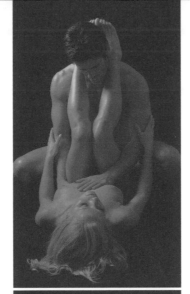
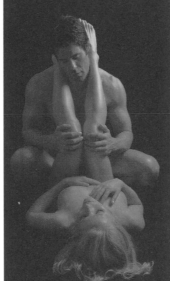
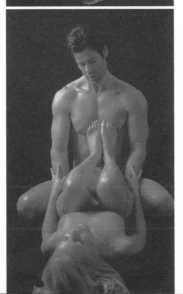

PURE KAMA SUTRA

DUNCAN BAIRD PUBLISHERS

LONDON

PURE

SEX SECRETS

KAMA

FOR MODERN LOVERS

SUTRA

NICOLE BAILEY

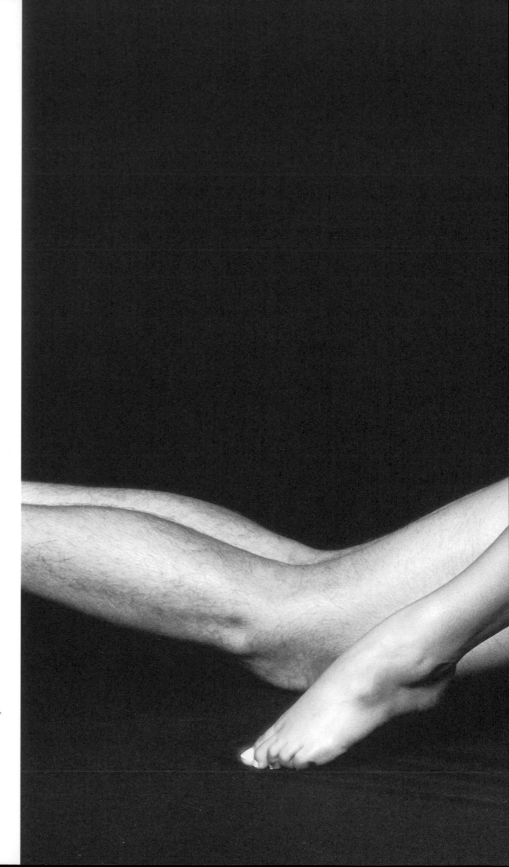

PURE KAMA SUTRA

NICOLE BAILEY

Distributed in the USA and Canada by
Sterling Publishing Co., Inc.
387 Park Avenue South, New York, NY 10016-8810

This edition first published in the UK and USA in 2005 by
Duncan Baird Publishers Ltd
Sixth Floor, Castle House, 75–76 Wells Street, London W1T 3QH

Managing Editor: Julia Charles
Editor: Zoë Stone
Managing Designer: Manisha Patel

Library of Congress Cataloging-in-Publication Data Available

ISBN-13: 978-1-84483-146-3

10 9 8 7 6 5 4

Typeset in Gill Sans
Color reproduction by Colourscan, Singapore
Printed in Hong Kong

For information about custom editions, special sales, premium and corporate
purchases, please contact Sterling Special Sales Department at 800-805-5489
or specialsales@sterlingpub.com.

PUBLISHERS' NOTE: The Publishers, the author and the photographer cannot
accept any responsibility for any injuries or damages incurred as a result of
following the advice in this book, or of using any of the techniques described
or mentioned herein. If you suffer from any health problems or special conditions,
it is recommended that you consult your doctor before following any practice
suggested in this book. Some of the advice in this book involves the use of
massage oil. However, do not use massage oil if you are using a condom – the
oil damages latex.

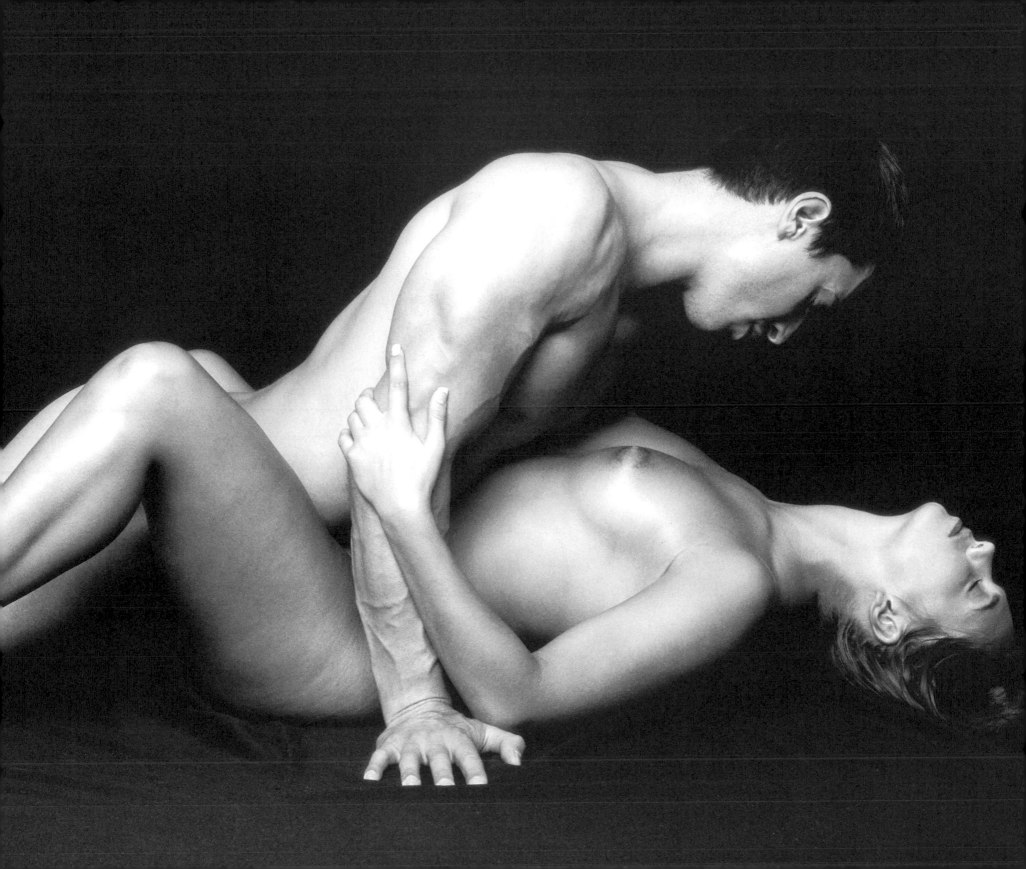

CONTENTS

INTRODUCTION

Mention the *Kama Sutra* and many people think of audacious lovemaking positions and exotic sex techniques. There's no doubt that the *Kama Sutra* contains both of these – but perhaps the most valuable lesson contained within its pages is that sex is a special occasion. Rather than relegating sex to the end of the day when you fall exhausted into bed – as many modern lovers do – the *Kama Sutra* treats sex as an important ritual. You prepare your environment, your body and your mind, and then – most importantly – you take time over sex. The *Kama Sutra* is good at paying attention to the fine details of lovemaking: the way you kiss, the way you nibble or scratch your lover's skin, even the angle and speed at which the penis moves inside the vagina.

WHAT IS THE *KAMA SUTRA*?

Very little is known about the man behind the *Kama Sutra*. His name is Vatsyayana Mallanaga and he is thought to have lived in India between 1 and 4CE. His collection of sutras (a sutra is an aphorism) was written in Sanskrit and takes the form of seven books. The word *kama* means pleasure, desire or sex.

Vatsyayana is believed to be the compiler of the *Kama Sutra* rather than its originator. His source was an array of existing Hindu erotic texts. Contrary to popular belief, only one of the seven *Kama Sutra* books is specifically about sex – the other six deal with the mores of erotic relationships, from guidelines about seducing a virgin to how to extract money from a lover.

Although the *Kama Sutra* is extremely old, it was unknown in the West until 1883. Sir Richard Francis Burton and his friend Forster Fitzgerald Arbuthnot were responsible for first translating it from Sanskrit into English. Publishing erotica – even ancient Indian literary erotica – was highly controversial in Victorian England, so Burton and Arbuthnot created their own publishing company, the Kama Shastra Society. Readers (mainly scholars and upper class gentlemen with a taste for erotica) bought the book by private subscription. In the 1960s the sexual revolution combined with the fashion for all things Indian meant that the English version of the *Kama Sutra* not only became acceptable but was celebrated for its sexual frankness. It was published formally in England and the United States in 1962.

THE *ANANGA RANGA* AND *THE PERFUMED GARDEN*

The Kama Shastra Society went on to publish two more Eastern love texts: The *Ananga Ranga* and *The Perfumed Garden*.

The *Ananga Ranga* was written originally in India in the 15th century by Kalyana Malla. Unlike the *Kama Sutra*, the whole of the *Ananga Ranga* is specifically about sex. Malla includes detailed lists of methods of embracing, kissing, scratching, biting and spanking, as well as positions for making love. Husbands were the intended readership and Malla's aim was to describe all the ways in which men could keep a marriage sexy.

The aim of *The Perfumed Garden* was also to stimulate and maintain passion, but for all men and women – not just those who were married to one another. Written by Sheikh Nefzawi in 16th-century Tunis, the text of *The Perfumed Garden* is considered more poetic, erotic and humorous in style than either the *Kama Sutra* or the *Ananga Ranga*. Its subjects include the characteristics of sexually desirable men and women, the ways in which to arouse a woman before sex, sex positions and exhaustive lists of the different types of male and female genitals.

PURE KAMA SUTRA

My book combines the wisdom of Vatsyayana, Kalyana Malla and Sheikh Nefzawi with modern insights into human sexuality. The emphasis is on making sex into a whole-body experience in which sensual pleasure ripples through your entire body, not just your genitals. The book is divided into five chapters: The Sensual Body, The Erotic High, Riding the Wave of Bliss, The Tantra of Ecstasy and The Undivided Self. Each chapter focuses on the practical – techniques that you can try with your lover right now.

In chapters 1 and 2, I describe how you and your lover can get in touch with each other sensually and erotically through methods such as genital massage and oral sex. Chapter 3 contains a selection of the most exciting and stimulating sex positions from the *Kama Sutra*, the *Ananga Ranga* and *The Perfumed Garden*. In chapters 4 and 5, I explain how you can take sex one step further than the physical realm. Through the ancient Indian practice of Tantra, and mindfulness, you and your lover can connect emotionally and spiritually and experience a unique sensation of oneness.

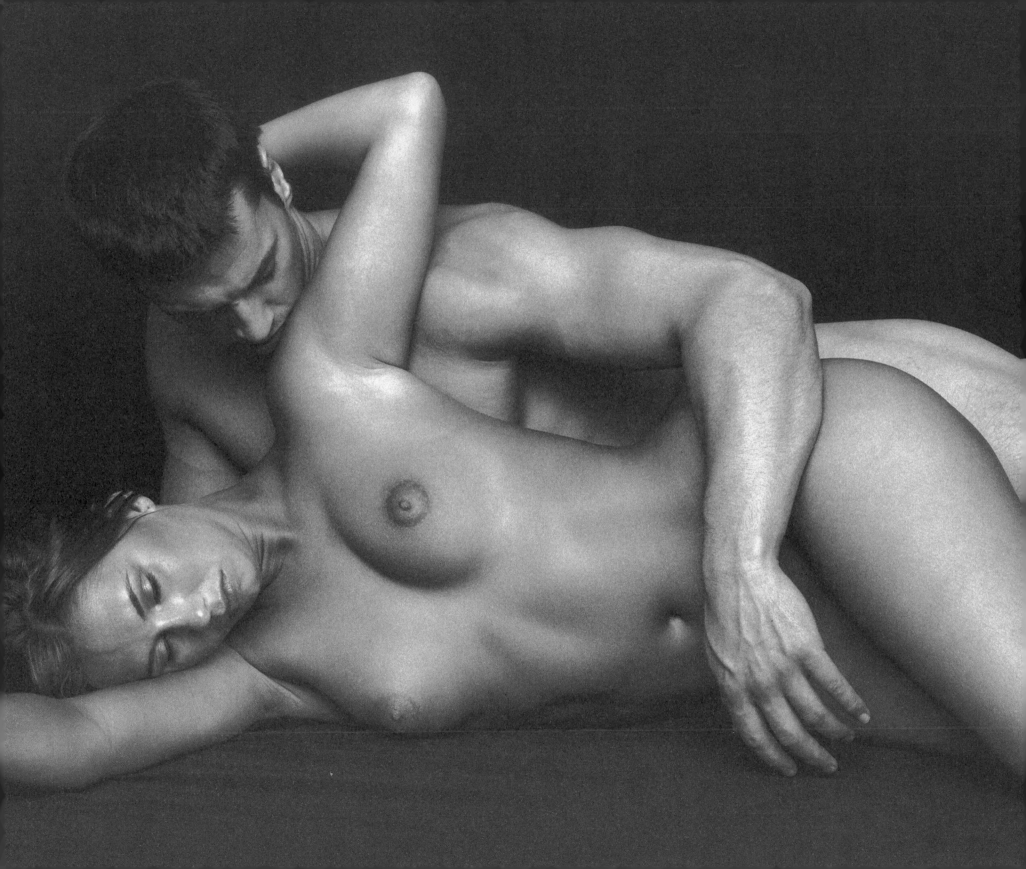

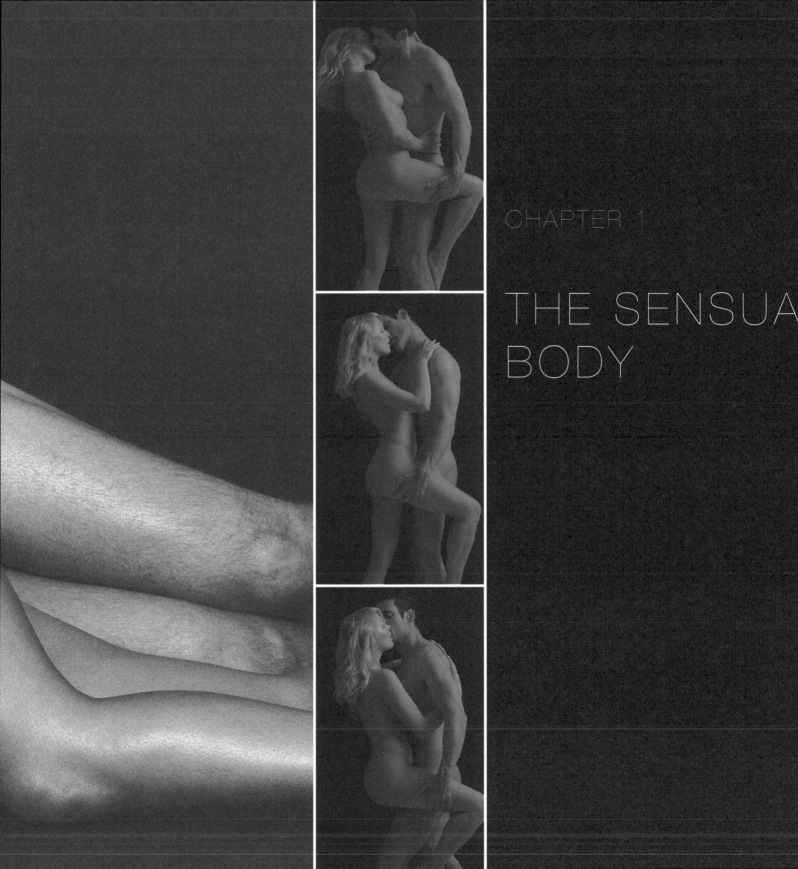

CHAPTER 1

THE SENSUA
BODY

EXPLORING THE SENSES

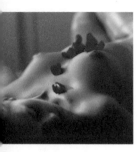

According to the *Kama Sutra*, foreplay should engage each of our five senses. The "pleasure room" should be fragrant with flowers and perfumes, the couple should drink, play musical instruments and talk together, then, as passion builds, they should touch and embrace one another's bodies.

Vatsyayana advocated that sex should have a strong ceremonial quality and, in his time, friends and servants had a specific role to play in the build-up to lovemaking: they helped the woman to bathe and dress and then brought refreshments for the couple. Finally when the lovers were overcome with lust, the servants were dismissed, but not before they had furnished the couple with flowers, ointments and betel leaves.

SEX-TIME

Attention to detail is something that is missing from many contemporary sex lives. If you tend to fall into bed at the end of the day and have perfunctory sex before falling asleep, set aside some special "sex-time". Imagine that you are preparing your bedroom for two people who are about to make love for the first time. Your job is to make the room appealing on many different levels — every detail matters. Think about the colour and texture of your bed linen. What looks sexy? What feels best against the skin? What about the lighting — will sex take place with the curtains open as the sun rises outside or at night time illuminated by candles? What music will you play — the sound of the sea, some fast, rhythmic drumming, or a love song?

The "pleasure room" should also smell sexy. Try burning incense or intoxicating essential oils such as jasmine or ylang ylang. In hot weather add a few drops of eucalyptus essential oil to water — it's great to spray on your skin when things get steamy. And think about taste too. Place chunks of mango and orange segments by the bed for you to suck on before kissing.

When you make love try switching the focus of your attention from one sense to another. If you usually concentrate on the sensation of your partner touching you, try thinking about what you see, taste, hear or smell during sex. See if you can become skilled at flicking from one sense experience to another in the way that you'd flick through television channels.

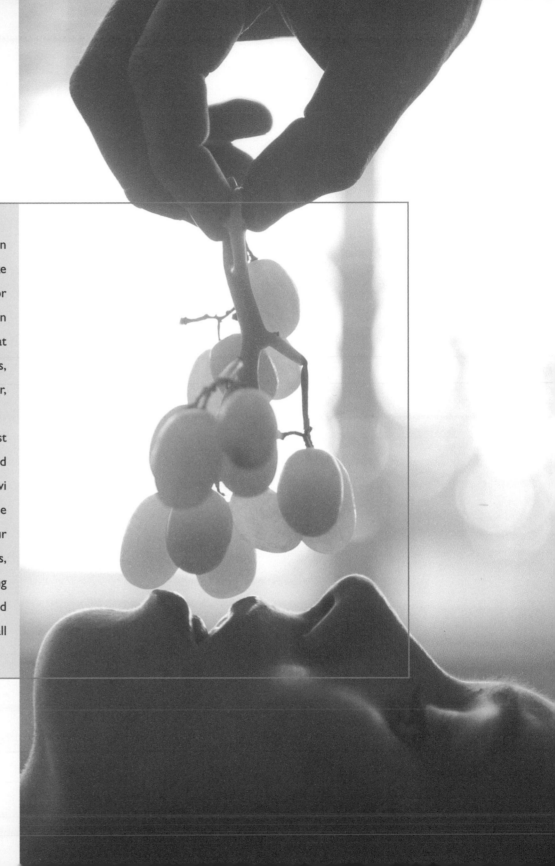

FOOD FOR THE SENSES

Sharing food with your lover can be a sexy, intimate or even sacramental act. First, choose some foods which you would like to feed to your lover and then sit down naked on the floor together. The aim is not to sate your appetite, but to reawaken your senses through food. Make sure that you select foods that have interesting textures, smells and tastes, such as asparagus, oysters, kiwi fruits, avocados, olives, honey, walnuts, caviar, cream and grapes.

Dispense with cutlery and use your fingers for the most sensual experience possible. Take your first piece of food and explore it together. For example, gently brush the skin of a kiwi fruit against your lover's lips, then split it open and inhale the fragrance of the flesh before letting the juice drip on to your tongues, down your chins and over your fingers. Some foods, such as frozen grapes or strawberries, are great for swapping between your mouths. When you have touched, tasted, smelled and observed each item of food in your collection, explore all the parts of each other's body in the same way.

THE SENSUAL TOUR

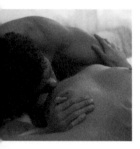

If you've been with a lover for a long time it's easy to get into sexual habits. Some of these might be good ones, such as telling a partner how beautiful or fantastic they are in bed, but others can prevent sex from being a whole-body experience. One of the most common bad sexual habits is to make a beeline for your partner's genitals shortly after you get into bed: after a brief kiss you start to stimulate his penis or her clitoris and as soon as he's hard and she's wet, you have intercourse. Of course, you can have fantastic sex like this, but just imagine what sex would be like if it lasted for hours and included not just your mouth, nipples and genitals, but also your ears, neck, belly, thighs, toes and all the other sensitive parts that tend to get ignored in the rush. As the *Kama Sutra* says, the man should caress the whole of the woman's body with his hands.

SLOW SEX

The sensual tour is a technique adapted from sex therapy. It's designed to slow sex down so that you can fully experience the sensations that you give and receive – like eating a gourmet meal incredibly slowly so that you can savour the taste of every bite. Making a sensual tour of each other's bodies is a great way to rediscover the art of eroticism and, if your sex life is in a rut, this is the way to reinvigorate it. One couple who tried the sensual tour spent the first hour stroking each other with a peacock feather, the second hour exchanging full-body massages with oils and the third hour on oral sex and intercourse.

Here are the guidelines for the sensual tour. Make sure that you have lots of time (a whole morning or afternoon if possible) and absolute privacy. Don't set out with the aim of reaching orgasm or having sex, just concentrate on touching each other in novel ways and in novel places. Focus on being playful, experimental and imaginative. Take turns to "tour" each other's body with your hands (or anything else!). As the giver of touch, your aim is to produce new and sensual sensations in your partner's body. As the recipient of touch, your aim is to immerse yourself in sensation and to give your partner feedback using words such as "harder", "softer" or "more" – or just a blissful "mmmm" if you've lost the ability to speak!

TOUCH TYPES

Use your hands, hair, feet, elbows, fingernails, teeth and tongue to stroke, caress and massage your lover's body. Experiment with different pressures; for example, your hands are extremely versatile – your fingertips can deliver a featherlight touch and your knuckles can produce deep static pressure. If you want to create the most subtle sensations imaginable, use your exhaled breath as a massage tool. Alternatively, lick a line along the nape of your lover's neck – or any other sensitive part of the body – and then blow along the length of that line.

You can also make a "toy box" of props, such as a silk scarf, a tennis ball and a string of beads, and use these to carry out touch experiments on your lover. Be imaginative: stroke each other's inner thighs with your fingernails, slide an ice-cube over her nipples, use a soft paintbrush to stroke his penis and balls, flick the tip of your tongue across the insides of her wrists or graze the tips of his fingers with your teeth. Massage parts of the body that you might not think of massaging: the ear lobes, the palms of the hands or along the line of the jaw.

SELF-MASSAGE

Being at home in your own body is one of the sexiest attributes that you can possess. Whether you are young or old, small or large, there is something powerfully attractive about being proud of your body. Apart from anything else you can enjoy the bliss of giving and receiving pleasure without feeling any inhibitions. If you don't possess it naturally, a sense of pride in your body isn't something that you can simply switch on. You need to work at it – and one of the best ways to do this is to learn how to touch your own body in a loving way.

MASSAGE TECHNIQUES

You don't have to attend massage classes to become an expert at self-massage. Just experiment with different forms of touch all over your body to find out what feels good to you. Try stroking your skin with the oiled flats of your palms, applying deep pressure with your thumbs or knuckles; grazing your skin with your fingernails; gently pinching, rubbing and squeezing your flesh between your thumb and fingers; or using a specially designed massage device or even a vibrator. Learn to give yourself a head

massage – use your fingertips in small, firm circles all over your head (so that your scalp moves) or gather fistfuls of your hair and make gentle, tugging movements. It also feels wonderful to apply pressure with the heels of your hands to the sensitive area above and in front of your ears.

More important than mastering specific techniques is to give yourself permission to experience pleasure solely by and for yourself. If you find yourself rushing through self-massage or thinking "this can't feel good because I'm doing it to myself", challenge yourself to lie back, relax and really take your time – give yourself up to sensation.

OILS AND LOTIONS

Self-massage feels best when your skin is silky smooth and your hands glide sensuously over your body with the minimum of friction. Spend time finding a lotion with a texture and a smell that you like. Even better than lotions are oils, because they stay on the surface of the skin for longer. You can use a base massage oil, such as sweet almond oil, but olive oil works just as well. For an aromatherapy massage, add a few drops of an essential oil such as jasmine or lavender to a carrier oil. Coconut oil is great if you're giving yourself a head massage – it also enhances the health of the hair and scalp.

SELF-PLEASURING

For many people the limit of their self-massage is masturbation. If this applies to you, resist the desire to make a beeline for your genitals. Imagine that you are trying to produce an orgasm in other parts of your body instead. Touch other erogenous areas such as your nipples, your neck, your inner thighs, your lips, your buttocks and your feet (see box, right). Can you feel aroused in parts of your body other than your genitals? Try to create a feeling of warmth, tingling, melting or shivering.

As sexual tension builds, try to hold on to it and savour it rather than dispersing it with a quick orgasm. When your whole body feels alive and responsive, start to stimulate your genitals slowly and mindfully, watching your arousal grow slowly toward the point of climax.

FEET FIRST

Soak your feet in warm water for around 15 minutes, then dry them and apply a generous amount of foot cream. Sit on a chair with one ankle resting on your opposite thigh. Now place your fingers on the top of your foot and apply deep, circular pressure to the base of your foot using your thumb. Massage the entire sole of your foot in this way. Now make your hand into a fist and apply pressure along the length of the sole of your foot using your knuckles.

Pay attention to your toes by taking each one in turn, pulling it up slightly and rolling it between your thumb and a finger. Then pinch and press the flesh between each toe.

Next, hold your ankle firmly in one hand and use the other hand to clasp your foot and rotate it in slow circles around your ankle. Release your foot and ankle and lightly pinch the flesh at the back of your ankle several times. To finish use the whole of your hand to gently stroke the length of your foot several times – both the top and the bottom. Repeat the massage on your other foot.

YONI MASSAGE

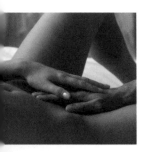

In the *Kama Sutra*, Vatsyayana recommends that a man should rub a woman's *yoni* (the Sanskrit word for vulva which means "sacred space") with his hands and fingers until it becomes soft – at which point he may put his *lingam* (penis) inside her. The importance of preparing a woman for sex is also stressed by Sheikh Nefzawi in *The Perfumed Garden*; a woman is compared to a fruit that releases its fragrance only when rubbed by the hands. Nefzawi says that the cleverest men are those who "take time to frolic" before lovemaking so that a woman can reach the highest enjoyment. Of course, contemporary lovers are aware that *yoni* massage isn't just a way of warming up women for intercourse; it's a type of sex in its own right. It is also effective after lovemaking when he has climaxed and she wants more.

IF YOU ARE THE GIVER

The secrets of a fantastic *yoni* massage are, first, to forget about time. Never clock-watch – tell yourself that there is absolutely nothing else that you should be doing at this moment. Second, treat the massage as a gift. Don't expect to receive anything on this occasion – just abandon yourself to the joy of giving. Third, communicate this joy by telling your lover how sexy or beautiful she looks or by moaning with pleasure yourself. Fourth, work with and respond to her body; match the rhythm of your fingers to the movements of her pelvis or the speed of her breathing. If you're not sure how she likes to be touched, ask her to put her fingers on top of yours to guide the pressure, speed and rhythm.

IF YOU ARE THE RECIPIENT

Sit or lie down in a position that feels comfortable and sexy. Many women choose to lie on their back, but you can also lie on your belly with your legs apart – this is a great position if you love having your buttocks nibbled, scratched, nuzzled or kissed – or sit in an armchair with your heels drawn up to your buttocks and your knees falling out to the sides. If it turns you on, watch what your lover is doing with his hands (if this is a major turn-on, set up a mirror so that you can see in detail). Alternatively, you might want to gaze into your lover's eyes, or close your eyes so that you can enter your own private world of erotic fantasy.

PLEASURING HER *YONI*

Coat your hands with massage oil and press one palm flat on your lover's vulva. Leave your hand there for about a minute to allow her to enjoy the sensation of warmth and pressure spreading slowly through her genitals and pelvis. Now use your hand to gently stroke the length of her from front to back. Use your fingers to massage and tweak her inner and outer labia (you can also gently tweak her pubic hair).

Now gently slide your longest finger into her vagina (as she becomes more aroused, you can insert more fingers). Explore the inside of her vagina by moving your finger(s) up and down and round and round. You can use your other hand to fondle her buttocks. Now withdraw your finger(s) and, without breaking contact, use your index finger to draw slow, gentle circles around the area of her clitoris. After a while alternate this with light flicking or tickling movements on her clitoris. Now put your finger(s) back in her vagina, but this time rest the pad of your thumb against her clitoris so that as you move your fingers in and out her clitoris is stimulated too.

LINGAM MASSAGE

As well as being the source of intense pleasure, the penis is also the source of much anxiety. Is it big enough? Will it get erect on demand? Will it stay erect? What if I come too soon? This is why the *lingam* (penis) massage is a fantastic and sexy treat to give to a man. The only thing that is required of him and his penis is to lie back and enjoy the sensations.

IF YOU ARE THE GIVER

If you usually stimulate your lover's penis to the point where he comes, change the emphasis of your touch. Even when your lover is highly aroused, resist the temptation to increase the speed or pressure of your massage strokes. Instead allow sexual arousal to go through a series of peaks and troughs. If your lover is about to ejaculate, you can dissipate his arousal in several ways. Don't echo your lover's body tension and/or rapid breathing. Instead make a conscious effort to relax and breathe deeply through your nose. This will encourage him to relax too. You can also take your hands away from his penis and stroke his belly or chest. Another time-honoured way of delaying ejaculation is to grasp his scrotum and gently pull down (the testicles get drawn up close toward the body when he's close to coming).

IF YOU ARE THE RECIPIENT

Get into a comfortable sitting or lying position. Focus on your breathing and turn your attention inward. As your lover stimulates your penis with her hands, let yourself enjoy the sensations without feeling any need to perform. You don't need to get a strong erection – or even any erection – you don't need to make love, and you don't need to come. If you have problems getting or keeping an erection, or ejaculating, this banishing of performance pressure can be extremely therapeutic.

Lingam massage is also good if you usually ejaculate very quickly. When you feel that you are reaching the point of no return, relax all the muscles in your body and concentrate on breathing deeply and evenly through your nose. You can also ask your lover to use methods to help you deplete your arousal (see above). With practice these techniques will give you the skill and confidence to help you control ejaculation during intercourse.

PLEASURING HIS *LINGAM*

Coat your hands in oil and gently rest one hand on his penis and testicles. Then enclose his penis in the palms of both hands. After a while, begin to roll his shaft gently between your palms. Then interlock your fingers and bring the heels of your hands together so that his penis is completely encircled by your hands. If his penis is long enough (or erect), rest the pads of your thumbs on his frenulum (this strip of skin that attaches the foreskin to the shaft is the hot spot of the penis).

Now tighten your grip and glide your interlocked hands along the length of his shaft and over the top of his glans. Make sure you have enough oil on your hands. Keep repeating this stroke using varying pressures and speeds – you can introduce a twisting motion if you like.

You can also try using the tip of your index finger to trace a line from the tip of his glans all the way down to his perineum and anus, or holding the base of his penis firmly in one hand while you use the pad of the thumb on your other hand to massage his frenulum in tiny circles.

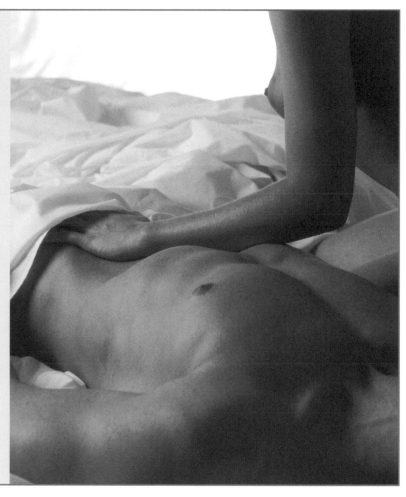

LOVE MUSCLES

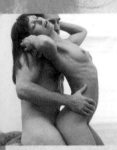

The most important muscles when it comes to sex are not your pecs, abs or biceps but your pelvic floor muscles – these are affectionately known as "love muscles". If you and your partner have both got fit, toned love muscles you will feel increased sensations during lovemaking – the vagina grips the penis tightly during sex, ejaculation can be delayed and the ripples of orgasm feel stronger for both of you.

In the *Kama Sutra* when a woman contracts her love muscles during sex it's known as the Mare's Position (see page 65) or the "pair of tongs". In the *Ananga Ranga* this technique is known as "constricting". The author of the *Ananga Ranga*, Kalyana Malla, states that the woman "must ever strive to close and constrict the *yoni* until it holds the *lingam*". With practice she will be able to squeeze the penis with her vagina in the same way that "the hand of the Gopala-girl milks a cow".

THE BIG SQUEEZE

The correct anatomical name for the love muscles are the pubococcygeal (PC) muscles. They occupy a triangle-shaped area

that stretches from the penis to the anus in men and the front of the vulva to the anus in women. These are the muscles that tend to be slacker and weaker after childbirth. For women the benefits of strong PC muscles are not just a better sex life but also a reduced chance of suffering from incontinence (leakage of urine) and uterine prolapse.

Men can locate their PC muscles by contracting the area around the penis and anus; women can locate their PC muscles by drawing up the area around the vagina and anus. You should feel a lifting sensation. If your muscles are weak, the sensation of lift slips away very quickly. This is a sure sign that your love muscles will benefit from a work-out. If you find it difficult to locate your PC muscles, attempt to stop urinating in mid-flow next time you go to the toilet – the muscles that you contract are your PC muscles.

Practise the exercises in the box (right) to get your PC muscles in shape to help you and your partner achieve heightened sensations during sex. Over time you may be able to fine-tune your muscle control to a high degree.

THE LOVE MUSCLE WORK-OUT

Squat down with your feet flat on the floor and your knees wide apart. If this is uncomfortable try sitting upright on a firm, flat seat. Now slowly draw up your love muscles until they are as fully contracted as possible. Hold this contraction for as long as you can – at first this may be only three seconds but over time you can build up to 10 seconds or more. Slowly release the contraction and let your muscles relax for 10 seconds. Now repeat the whole exercise up to 10 times.

You may find it helpful to visualize the contraction as an elevator that slowly rises and descends through a series of floors – say three to start with. Imagine that you are going to stop the elevator for a few seconds at each of the three floors, both on the upward and the downward journey. Then, as you develop greater muscle control, add more floors.

Try a second exercise known as the fast squeeze. Instead of contracting your muscles slowly, as you did in the last exercise, draw them up rapidly and release them rapidly. Try to perfect a fast and rhythmic pumping action.

HOW TO USE HER LOVE MUSCLES DURING SEX

Once you have practised contracting your PC muscles and you have good control of them, try massaging your lover's penis by alternately relaxing and contracting them during sex. If you've got really fine muscular control, you may able to "flutter" your muscles against his penis. Try contracting your muscles to their full "height" during the build-up to orgasm. Experiment to find the level of tension that feels good.

HOW TO USE HIS LOVE MUSCLES DURING SEX

With practice you can use your PC muscles to stop yourself ejaculating. This way if you are feeling very aroused, you can pull back from orgasm and make sex last as long as you and your partner want it to. As you feel yourself building up to ejaculation, contract your PC muscles as strongly as you can and breathe deeply. Some men can refine this muscle control to the point where they can experience the contractions of orgasm without actually ejaculating – this enables them to go on making love and even experience multiple orgasms.

OPENING THE BODY

Sometimes all the ingredients for perfect sex are there – you're passionately in love with your partner, you've got a whole evening ahead of you and there's nothing else to do or think about apart from pure, uninterrupted sex. Yet when it comes to it, the feelings you experience during foreplay and intercourse aren't as powerful as they could be.

BODY ARMOUR

Many people hold tension in their bodies and specifically their genitals. Tension is usually thought of as being physical in origin, but it can also be emotional. Negative experiences such as bad or disappointing sexual encounters can be "stored" in the pelvic area with the result that the lower part of the body becomes less responsive to pleasurable touch. For example, imagine a woman who habitually feels close to climaxing, but never quite gets the right stimulation to tip her over the edge into orgasm. In the long term her body is likely to stop responding to touch so that even when she gets the stimulation she needs to orgasm she can no longer "feel" these sensations.

FREEING THE BODY

There are two principal ways to free the body from emotional and physical tension so that you are able to experience sexual pleasure as fully and deeply as possible. The first is massage, which can have a profoundly healing effect on the body. Try the genital massages on pages 18–21. The second is movement – by moving and stretching the hips, groin and pelvic area, you release any tension and get energy in these areas flowing again.

The three exercises on the following pages are designed to free and invigorate the lower body. They are postures from the Indian tradition of Hatha yoga and are easy enough for anyone to try. A positive side effect of all of the postures is that they increase strength and suppleness in your lower body and as a result you'll find many of the sex positions in Chapter 3 a lot easier to get into!

As you do each posture, bring your awareness to your breathing and try to cultivate the art of directing your breath into your pelvis and genitals (you can do this using visualization; see page 141). Imagine that each breath has healing properties.

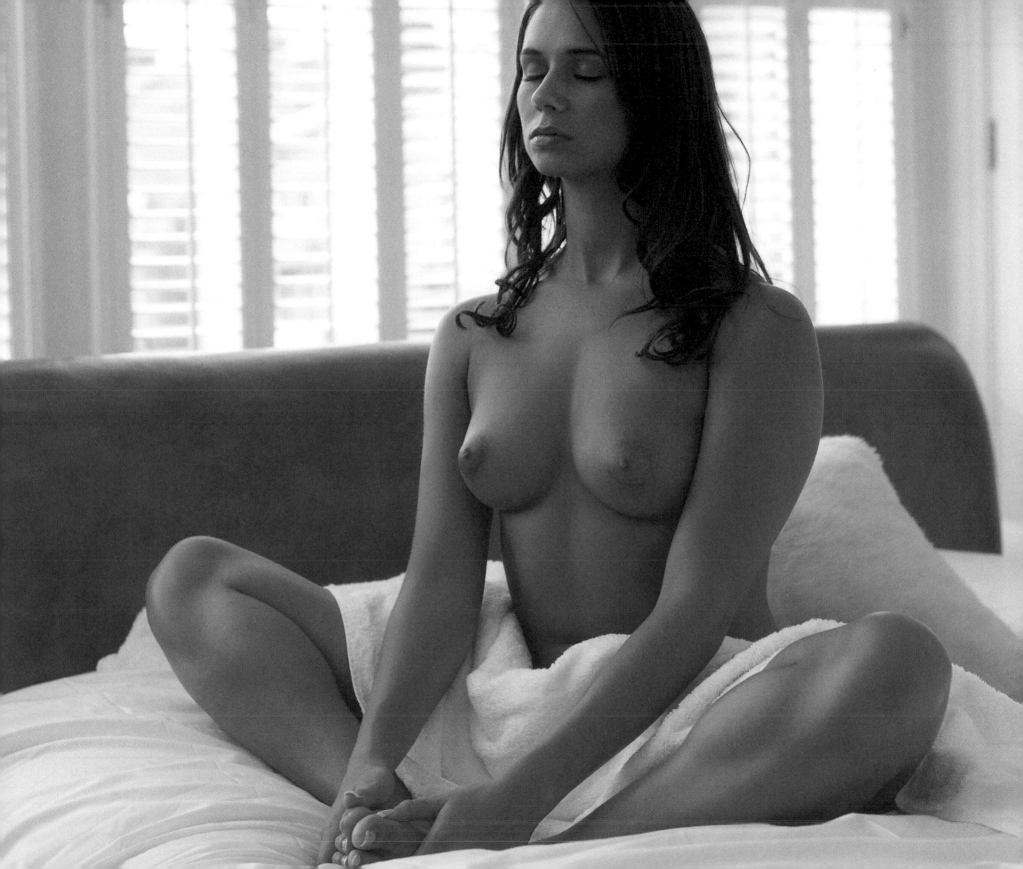

Become aware of the subtle sensations in your hips, pelvis and genitals and experiment within each posture. For example, how does it feel if you contract your love muscles (see page 22) during the Butterfly Pose?

BUTTERFLY POSE

Sit on the floor – don't slump, but don't arch your back inward either. Bring the soles of your feet together and place your hands on your feet or shins. Your feet should be close enough to your body to produce some amount of tension in your groin area, but not so close that it feels uncomfortable. Keep your back long and straight. Without moving your feet see if you can get your knees to drop a little lower by consciously relaxing and opening your groin area (directing your breath into your hips and groin area can help you to achieve this).

Slowly at first, now bounce your knees up and down. Imagine your groin becoming more elastic and open, and any tension just melting away. Bounce your knees faster. Experiment with the speed and depth of the bounces – for example,

alternate between a fast flutter and a deep, slow movement (imagine that you are flapping a very heavy pair of wings).

Sit still for a few moments before folding forward at your hips as though you are aiming to touch your feet with your chest. Keep a straight back. Then sit upright and close your eyes for a few moments before slowly standing up.

BRIDGE POSE

Lie on your back with your arms by your sides and take a few moments to relax. Bend your knees and place your feet flat on the floor hip-width apart. Lift your hips off the floor and draw your arms underneath your lower back or your bottom. Link your hands together and push your pelvis as high as you can. Breathe deeply. Observe the sensations in your thighs, groin and abdomen. Imagine these areas opening up.

Move in and out of Bridge Pose by repeatedly lowering and lifting your body. When you lower your body, your buttocks should just touch the floor (or your linked hands). Try to move in a smooth, undulating movement – as well as freeing up the pelvis, this movement can be deeply sensual, especially if you do it in time to a piece of music. Observe the different sensations you experience when you practise the same motion with your legs spread wide apart.

When you want to stop, lie flat on the floor and stretch your legs out. Bring your knees up to your chest and hug them with your arms. Keep your head on the floor and rock gently from side to side (this will gently massage the muscles in your back). This is a counterpose that stretches your spine in the opposite direction to the Bridge Pose.

HIP OPENER

Sit on the floor with your legs out straight in front of you. Keep your back straight and tall, bend your right leg and draw it across the front of your body so that your knee rests in the crook of your right elbow and your foot rests in the crook of your left elbow. Hug your leg to your chest with your hands joined on the outside of your calf. If you find this difficult, just hold your knee and foot with your hands instead. Concentrate on releasing tension from your hip area. Hold the pose for the length of five deep breaths and then relax. Alternatively, you can rock your leg gently from side to side five times (as though you are rocking a baby) to open up your hips even more. Repeat the posture with your other leg. If you find it hard to keep your back straight, try doing the exercise while lying flat on your back.

This posture is an excellent preparation for the yoga position in which you tuck each foot into the hip socket of the opposite leg – the lotus. And if you are a woman and have mastered the lotus, you and your partner can try having sex in the Lotus Position on pages 74–5.

CLOSING RELAXATION

After doing yoga it's a good idea to spend a brief period of time relaxing to give your body a chance to assimilate the benefits of the postures. Lie on your back with your legs apart and your arms a little way away from your body. Alternatively, you and your partner can sit back-to-back on the floor. Close your eyes and tune in to the ebb and flow of your breath for a few minutes.

PREPARING THE BODY

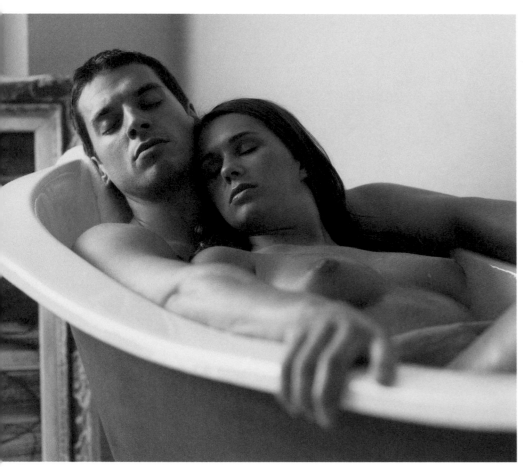

The *Kama Sutra* is hot on personal hygiene. Vatsyayana describes the care that a man should take of his body: he should bathe daily, anoint his body with oil every other day, cover his body with lather every third day, and shave his head and face every fourth day. He should be scrupulous about washing his teeth and armpits. Perfumes and ointments may be worn in moderation and the lips may be coloured with a substance called *alactaka*. Removal of all body hair is recommended every five to ten days.

GETTING INTO YOUR BODY

One of the benefits of cleaning and pampering rituals is that they bring you back into your body and help you to relax; two essential pre-requisites for great sex. Having a pre-sex bath or shower (see box, opposite) isn't just about feeling clean, it's also about getting rid of stress. The aim is to leave the bathroom and enter the bedroom feeling fresh in both mind and body.

How you relax your mind and get into your body before sex is entirely up to you. You can take the tried and trusted route of bathing or you may like to try something more unorthodox,

CLEANSING THE MIND AND BODY

Set an alarm (one that sounds gentle rather than intrusive) to ensure that you take a full 30-minute pre-sex bath or shower. Really savour the experience – this is time by and for yourself.

Get in your bath or shower, close your eyes and slowly count to 100. Concentrate on the feeling of water on your body. If you are standing in the shower, lift your face to the jets of water and feel them pummel your skin. If you are in a bath, feel the water enveloping your body like a glove; sink below the water-level for a few moments and relish the feeling of immersion.

Now take a virtual tour of your body starting with your feet and working upward to the crown of your head. Which parts of your body feel hot or cold? How does the water feel against your belly, your back, your genitals or your hands? Is there any tension in your body? If you are in a shower can you direct the stream of water onto the points of tension?

Once you get out stand still for a few moments feeling the water dripping and running down your body – allow yourself to shiver a little before wrapping yourself in a warm towel.

such as applying temporary tattoos or body paint in unusual places, or giving yourself a sensual foot massage. Some people like to exercise before sex – the feeling of being fit, alive and invigorated can be the ultimate turn-on. Research backs this up: bursts of exercise boost the male sex hormone testosterone.

TURN UP THE SMELL

Body smells are important during sex – something that both ancient and modern sex manuals will verify. No-one wants to smell stale sweat on their lover's body, but many people cleanse themselves so thoroughly that not a trace of their own body smell remains. Fresh sweat contains chemicals known as pheromones that act as powerful natural attractants. Think of the sensation you feel when someone smells "right" to you – it's not their perfume or aftershave, but something far more subtle and indefinable that draws you close and makes you want to breathe that person in. So if you habitually bathe before sex, try washing with water alone to allow your natural fragrance to shine through without being overshadowed by cosmetic smells.

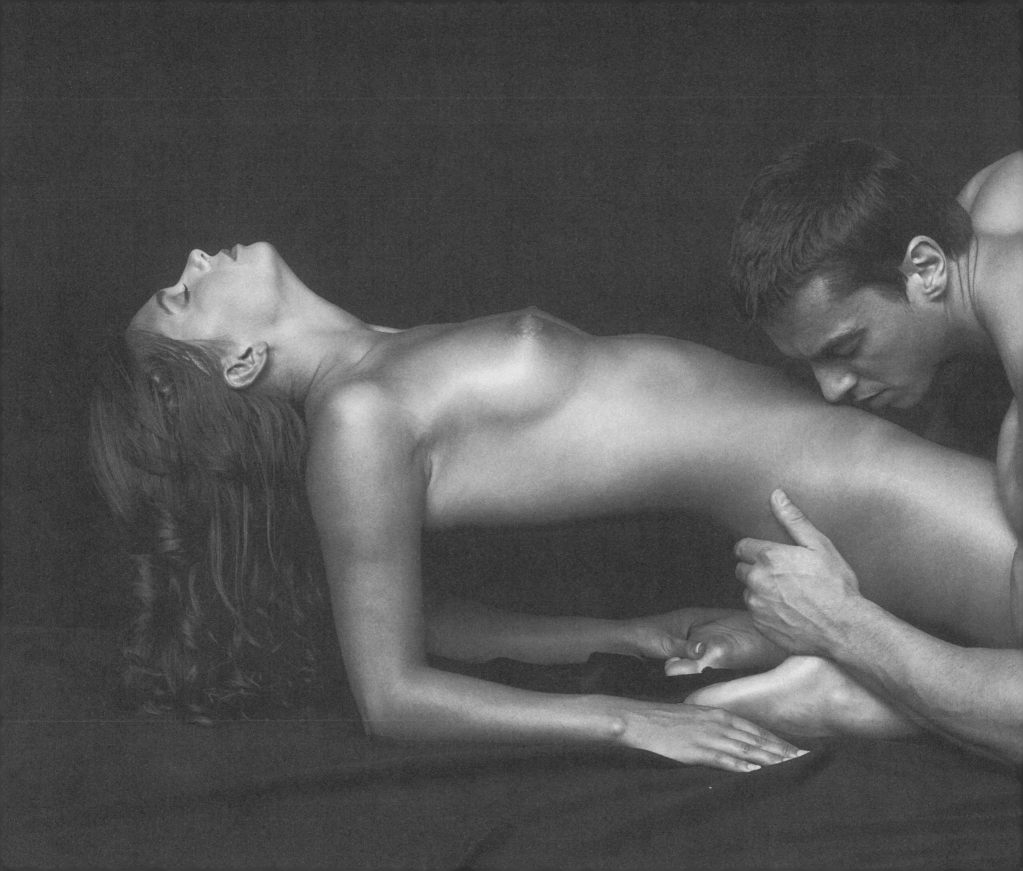

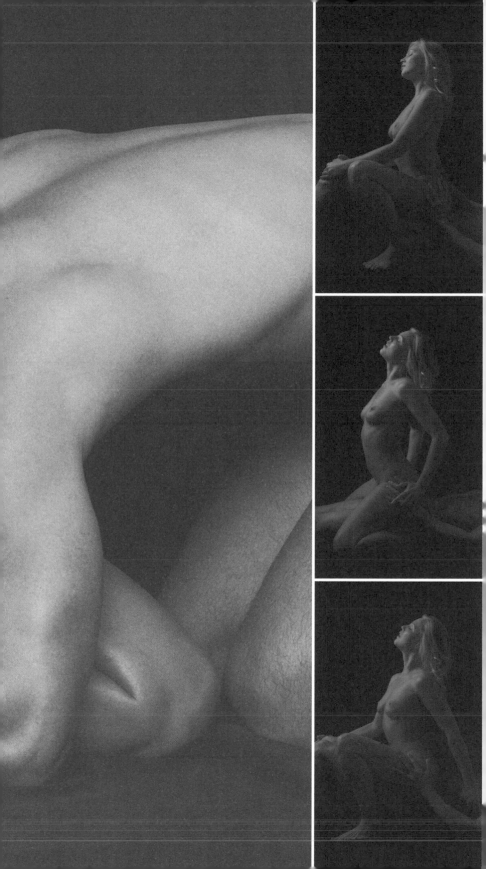

SEX GAMES AND ADVENTURES

The women of the harem in Vatsyayana's *Kama Sutra* were permitted to pleasure themselves with bulbs, roots and fruits that "took the form of the *lingam*". They were also allowed to lie down upon the erect *lingam* of a male statue. But apart from these improvised sex aids, little mention is made of toys and games in the *Kama Sutra*. In contrast contemporary lovers can draw upon a massive range of sex props and ideas to make sex into adult playtime.

TOYS FOR GROWN-UPS

Whether it's a vibrator, nipple clamp, anal plug, penis ring or feather duster, there's bound to be a sex toy that engages your curiosity. The range of sex toys available is huge – especially if you shop online. The problem is not finding something that appeals to you, but sustaining interest in a sex toy once you have it – many quickly lose their novelty value. It helps to give sex toys a partial role in sex rather than making them the main feature. For example, use a vibrator on each other during foreplay or on her clitoris during intercourse, but not both. Alternatively, use sex toys occasionally and build them into imaginative role-playing scenes. For example, if you are playing master and slave, the slave can have a box of tools (such as vibrators and fur-lined paddles) dedicated to pleasing his or her master.

PLAYING THE PART

If you've ever fantasized about making love with a different person or even *being* a different person during sex, role-playing is for you. Couples often say that role-playing is a good way to overcome aspects of sex that they feel inhibited about. For example, if you feel uncomfortable talking dirty during sex, pretending that you're someone else by dressing up, talking and acting in character releases you from all of your usual feelings of self-consciousness. Role play can be serious, funny or facetious; both of you or just one of you can adopt a persona.

During role play you can take on any character you choose – the traditional characters for sexual role play include doctor and nurse (or doctor and patient), nun and vicar, school girl and headmaster, and slave and master. But you can use your

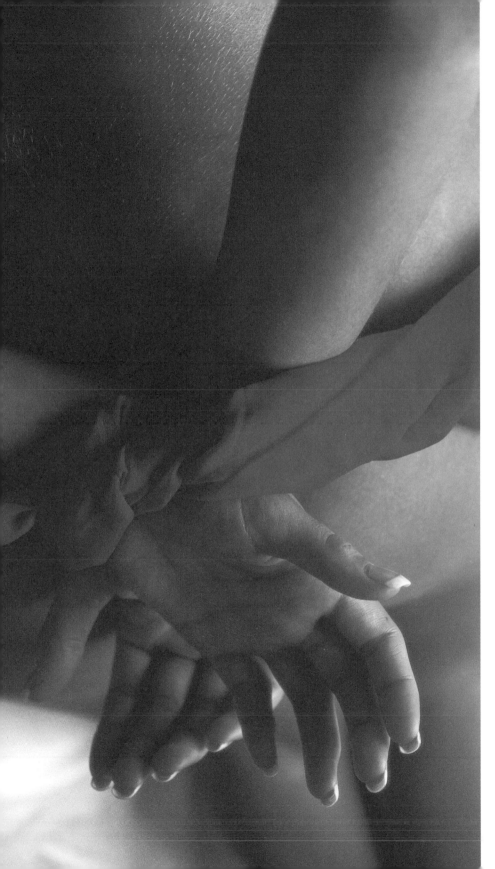

imagination to go beyond these stereotypes. Become whoever or whatever you like – you can be animals rather than humans if you want to! Even the simple act of speaking in a different accent or inventing new names for each other during sex can inspire you to act in novel ways.

If role playing works for you and your lover, go as far as you can to create realistic roles. Pay attention to the details – as well as dressing and speaking in character, adopt the body language, facial mannerisms and sexual habits of your alter ego.

A LITTLE LIGHT BONDAGE

Tying up your lover instantly puts you in charge of a sexual encounter and him or her in a position of extreme vulnerability. If you completely trust one another, bondage can be a great way to explore issues of power and submission – some couples say that bondage games take them to unprecedented heights of arousal. Even if you feel self-conscious during other types of role-playing games, there's something about physical restraint that makes it easy to slip into character.

Technique is important in bondage games – as the restrainee you want to be taken seriously, but you don't want to hurt your lover. Use stockings, tights, silk scarves, leather or rubber straps, or thick soft rope. As always in sexual games, if something hurts, stop. If you develop a taste for bondage, sex shops stock a vast array of restraining equipment from chains and handcuffs to collars and leads.

Consider to which object you will tie your lover – for example, the bed posts, a chair or even a shower head – or whether you will simply bind their wrists or ankles. Decide also whether you want to increase their powerlessness by using a blindfold. It also helps to have an approximate idea of what you are going to do to your lover – if you seem assured of your moves, this adds to the authenticity of your role. For example, you could tease your lover by undressing slowly and provocatively, pausing occasionally to kiss them, then giving them oral sex until they are close to orgasm. Aim for a drawn-out sexual encounter in which you tease, tantalize, arouse and withdraw from your partner in repeating cycles.

SPEED-WRITE A FANTASY

Try this exercise with your lover. Sit down with a pen and paper each and write down three sexual fantasies as fast as you can. Speed is important here – the more time you have, the more likely you are to process and modify your thoughts before you get them down on paper. It's a good idea to have a stopwatch and allow yourself no more than two or three minutes per fantasy. Don't plan what you're going to write in advance, instead write in a stream-of-consciousness style in which you don't judge or censor your thoughts. Your ideas can be as wild and risqué or loving and romantic as you want them to be.

Try to let go of your inhibitions with each narrative you write. You may find that the third one you write is the most honest, adventurous or compelling. At the end of the exercise, you can swap pieces of paper with your lover or read your ideas aloud to each other. If you don't feel comfortable doing this, just discuss the themes that have come up. Next talk to your lover about whether you would like to enact any of your desires and how you could go about doing this.

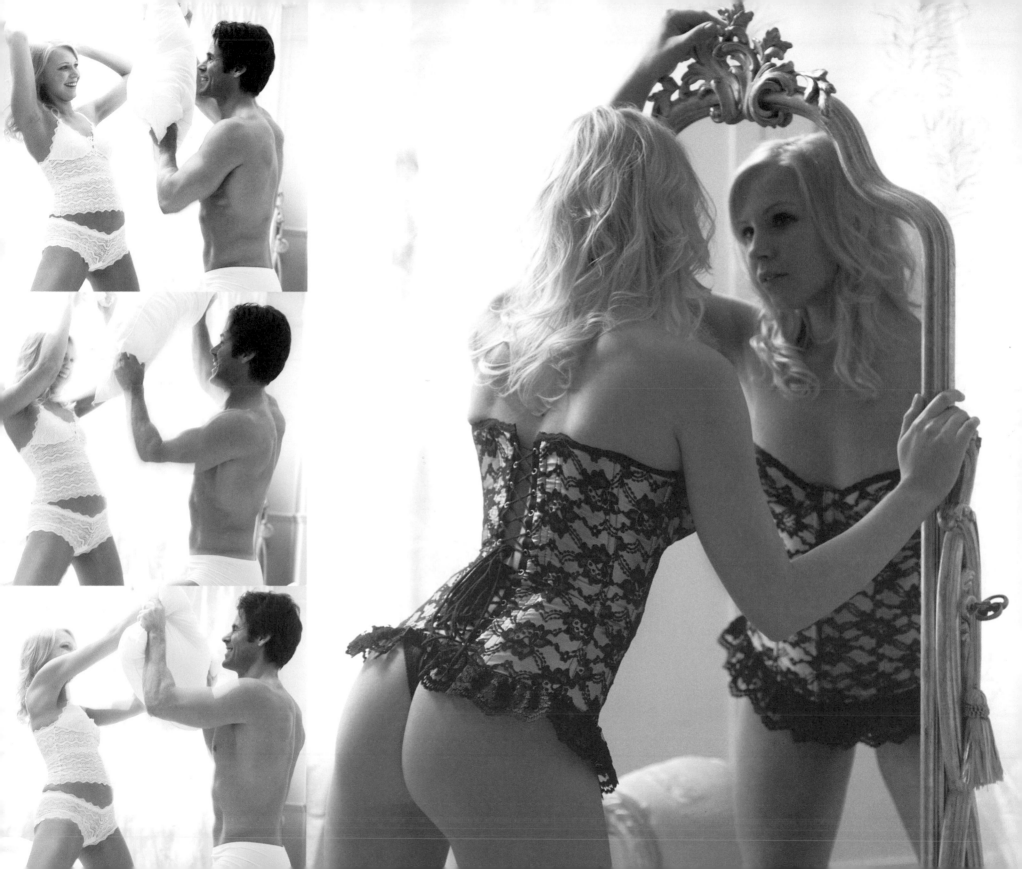

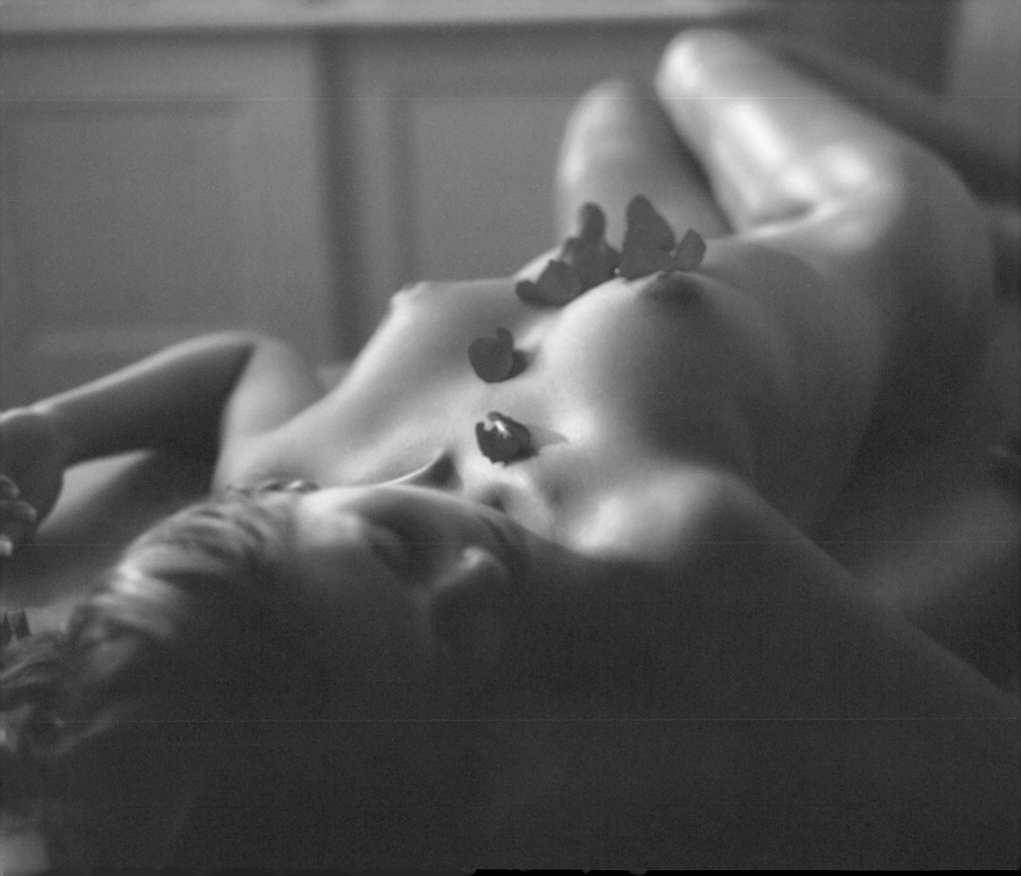

THE SEXUAL WISH-LIST

At some point many people have wished for an adventurous sex life. Creating a sexual wish-list is a fun way of communicating your wildest sexual dreams to your lover. It's also a good follow-up to writing your own fantasies (see box, page 34) because you can include some of these ideas in your wish-list. Do the following exercise together with your lover and use these categories in your list:

Venue: write down the places in which you dream of making love, these can be anywhere from a forest to a hotel balcony.

Games: describe any roles that you would like to play with your lover during sex.

Novel Acts: if there's something sexual that you've never tried and want to, such as filming yourself during sex, trying out a new sex toy or even having a threesome, write it down.

Talking: write down your aspirations about sexual communication. This could mean anything from wanting to talk more frankly about your sex life with your lover to wanting to talk dirty during intercourse.

SEDUCTIVE DANCING

Dancing brings you in touch with your body, releases inhibition and is a huge turn-on. Treat it as a form of foreplay. Play a piece of music that you both love, and dance together. Start by dancing around each other, so that you are close but not touching. Try not to break eye contact. As the sexual tension mounts, let your bodies touch, and begin to dance in synchrony. Dance back to back, front to back and finally front to front. When the music stops, stand very still and immerse yourself in the sensation of your lover's body pressed against yours.

The sexiest dances happen when you move the whole of your body. Forget about following carefully choreographed steps and instead make up your own movements. You can dance to any type of music you like, from romantic ballads through pop songs to classical music. Some people find that they can really lose themselves when dancing to tribal music; choose something that has a rhythmic, repetitive quality, such as drumming or chanting. Close your eyes and try to let your body absorb the sound so that you begin to feel connected to the music.

KISSING, BITING AND SCRATCHING

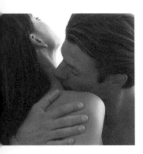

The author of *The Perfumed Garden*, Sheikh Nefzawi, believes that sharing a truly intense kiss is like lighting a fire that can be extinguished only by sex. Kissing is not only one of the most potent types of stimulation there is, Nefzawi says, but it also generates a uniquely sweet and delicious type of saliva that is more intoxicating than the strongest wine and can cause men to experience whole body shivers. He states that kissing should always be passionate, describing brief kisses that are delivered to the outside of the lips as useless and meant only for children! A real kiss requires wet lips and involves your tongues dancing in and out of each other's mouth. The *Ananga Ranga* follows the same premise: the author, Kalyana Malla, gives an example of one of the most erotic kisses – the woman should cover her lover's eyes with her hand, shut her own eyes and thrust her tongue in and out of his mouth in a way that's evocative of the penis sliding in and out of the vagina.

Contemporary lovers know that it's not only the kissing technique that is important but also how often you kiss. Truly passionate mouth-to-mouth kisses often get deprioritized by couples who've been together for a long time. If this applies to you, put kissing back at the top of your sexual agenda. Kiss frequently and for long periods, and kiss for the sheer heady pleasure of it. Give your lover a deep tongue kiss as you're saying goodbye and then walk away feeling so aroused that you can't wait for the moment you're together again.

MARKING THE BODY

Nothing inflames a sense of love so much as marks left on the body, says Vatsyayana (the author of the *Kama Sutra*). Scratches and bites act as a physical reminder of sex. They are stamps of sexual ownership and some lovers wear them with a great sense of pride. Times for marking the body, says Vatsyayana, are when a lover is going away (or returning) or when angry lovers are reconciled. In the *Ananga Ranga* the word *kolacharcha* is the name given to the deep and lasting bite marks given by a man to a woman when he is going to a foreign land – after his disappearance the woman will look at the marks and remember her husband with a yearning heart.

MAKING YOUR MARK

Body marks are entirely a matter of personal taste – you may think they're sexy and evocative or maybe you just can't see the appeal. If you want to try some of Vatsyayana's suggestions, make sure that your teeth and nails are clean and smooth – your aim is to apply a small amount of pressure and create novel sensations, not to break the skin or cause pain. Ask your lover's permission first. The following techniques are from the *Kama Sutra* and the *Ananga Ranga*:

Sounding: gently drag your nails across the surface of your lover's skin to make their body hair stand up and give them goose bumps.

The Half Moon: gently press your nails into your partner's buttocks to create temporary half-moon shapes.

The Coral and the Jewel: this technique is also known as the love bite. Draw the flesh of your lover's neck into your mouth by sucking; now very gently nibble with your teeth.

Prasritahasta: keep your palm open and your hand relaxed and pat or spank your lover's buttocks.

MOUTH CONGRESS

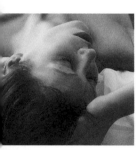

Receiving genital kisses, licks and sucks is the ultimate in sexual sensation for many men and women. Vatsyayana calls it "mouth congress"; we know it as oral sex or simply "going down".

FORBIDDEN PLEASURES

Some of the pleasure of oral sex comes from the fact that it retains its aura of the forbidden, despite it being widely talked about and practised. Oral sex has been frowned upon in the past and still is today in some cultures. For example, although the *Kama Sutra* provides details of oral sex techniques, Vatsyayana claims that oral sex opposes the moral code and dismisses it as a low practice that is performed only by eunuchs, unchaste and wanton women, female attendants, and serving maids.

CONGRESS OF A CROW

The 69 (or "Congress of a Crow" as it is called in the *Kama Sutra*) in which you both lick and suck each other at the same time is a matter of preference – it can drive you wild with pleasure or wild with frustration (because neither of you get the right amount of detailed attention). But if the 69 is your position of choice, there are several variations: him on his back with her on top (or vice versa), both of you lying on your sides with your heads resting on each other's inner thigh, and the most athletic position of all – the standing 69. To get into this position, the woman lies on her back with her head off the edge of the bed – the man stands astride her head and then leans over her body and picks her up so that his mouth is opposite her genitals. Try this as a quickie novelty position (but bear in mind that it's only really viable if she is light).

MOUTH CONGRESS FOR HER

Mouth congress for women doesn't receive much attention in the *Kama Sutra*, although Vatsyayana says that some women of the harem may perform "acts of the mouth" on each other's *yonis*. Yet oral sex is a great pre- or post-intercourse act that many women relish as an intimate and erotic gift.

There's no right or wrong way to give cunnilingus – everyone's different – but if you're the giver, help her to get into

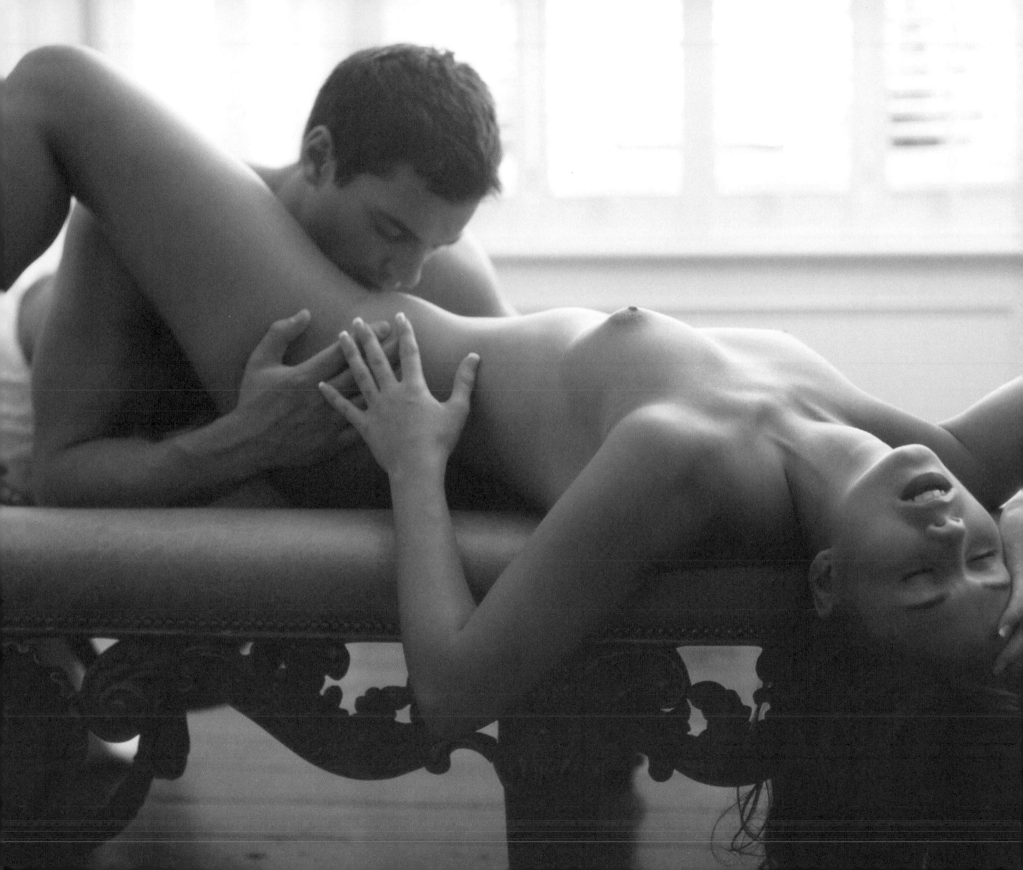

MOUTH STROKES FOR HER

Experiment with these strokes. Ask her for plenty of feedback about what she enjoys. Alternatively, ask her to lick or suck the tip of your little finger in the way that she would like you to stimulate her clitoris.

• Make your tongue hard and flick the tip side to side or back and forth on her clitoris.

• Press your lips around her clitoral hood – now suck. At the same time, use your tongue to flick, lick or stroke her clitoris.

• Make your tongue relaxed and flat, and make broad tongue strokes across the entire clitoral area.

• Use the point of your tongue to draw circles around her clitoris – start slowly then speed up.

• Put your first two fingers flat on either side of her clitoral hood and then squeeze them together to push her clitoris up and out. Now very gently lick her clitoris.

• Use your tongue on her clitoris while you insert your longest fingers into her vagina and massage her G-spot (see pages 46–7). Do this all the way to orgasm.

a relaxed, sensual state first. You can do this by caressing and kissing her feet and then moving your way up her legs massaging and stroking them as you go. When you go down on her, show your appreciation by telling her how beautiful she looks, smells or tastes. And it may sound obvious but the clitoris is the epicentre of erotic pleasure so concentrate your attention here rather than on the vagina. If you want to stimulate her vaginally at the same time, you can massage her G-spot with your fingers or a vibrator. Once you've started cunnilingus, keep going, stay focused and don't let your attention drift! Aim to find the strokes that she really loves and keep that rhythm going.

POSITIONS FOR CUNNILINGUS

The first rule of oral sex is be comfortable, especially if she wants to come. Some oral sex positions, such as her kneeling or squatting over his face, can be great turn-ons, but difficult to hold for any length of time. If you're the recipient, find a position that works for you: try lying back on a big pile of cushions or pillows and letting your legs fall to the sides or sitting on the edge of the bed or armchair and lying back. Other positions, such as her standing and him kneeling, are enjoyable but it can be hard for him to apply his lips and tongue in exactly the way she needs.

MOUTH CONGRESS FOR HIM

Men love oral sex and most men would like more than they get. This was the conclusion of sex writer Susan Crain Bakos who asked more than 1,000 men whether they received as much oral sex as they wanted. 75 per cent of them answered "no".

Many men say that fellatio is an intense form of pleasure because the mouth can deliver an amazing array of pressures and sensations – more so than the vagina – and men are free during oral sex to lie back and enjoy themselves without any distractions or pressure to perform. For some men, such as Seth (quoted in Nancy Friday's *Men in Love*), fellatio is a favourite fantasy: "I imagine she sucks all of me at once; simultaneously devouring both my penis and balls. After ejaculation she tenderly sucks until my penis is drained and limp. We embrace and kiss. It is a long, drawn-out kiss and we are satisfied."

MOUTH STROKES FOR HIM

These eight oral sex techniques all come from the *Kama Sutra* and are designed to be performed one after the other:

Nominal Congress: hold his penis in your hand and caress the top with your lips and tongue.

Biting the Sides: hold the tip of his penis with your fingers and nuzzle and nibble the sides of his shaft.

Outside Pressing: press your lips around his glans in a tight seal and move your mouth up and down, sucking as you do so.

Inside Pressing: take as much of his penis into your mouth as you can, press your lips tightly around his shaft and then hold for a moment before pulling away.

Kissing: hold his penis in your hand and cover it with kisses using your lips and tongue, as if you are kissing his lower lip.

Rubbing: lick his penis; swirl your tongue around his glans.

Sucking a Mango Fruit: enclose the top half of his penis in your mouth and suck.

Swallowing It Up: take as much of his penis into your mouth as you can and suck – imagine swallowing up his penis.

What's clear from men's descriptions of oral sex is that there's no single right way to perform fellatio. For example, some men enjoy licks and gentle nibbles, others enjoy lots of head movement and strong suction and others like a combination of simultaneous hand and mouth action.

TECHNIQUES OF THE EUNUCHS

A technique used by eunuchs in the *Kama Sutra* to heighten the sense of the forbidden during oral sex can be revived and used by modern lovers. When the eunuch discovers that his client has an erection he chastises him for becoming aroused and only begins mouth congress after much protestation. He then performs eight oral sex techniques (see box, page 43) in sequence, pausing at the end of each one to express his reluctance to continue. Only after much persuasion does he relent and take his client's penis back into his mouth. Scolding a partner for becoming aroused and expressing false reluctance to stimulate them are classic role-playing techniques – try them out and see if you can drive your lover to new heights of arousal.

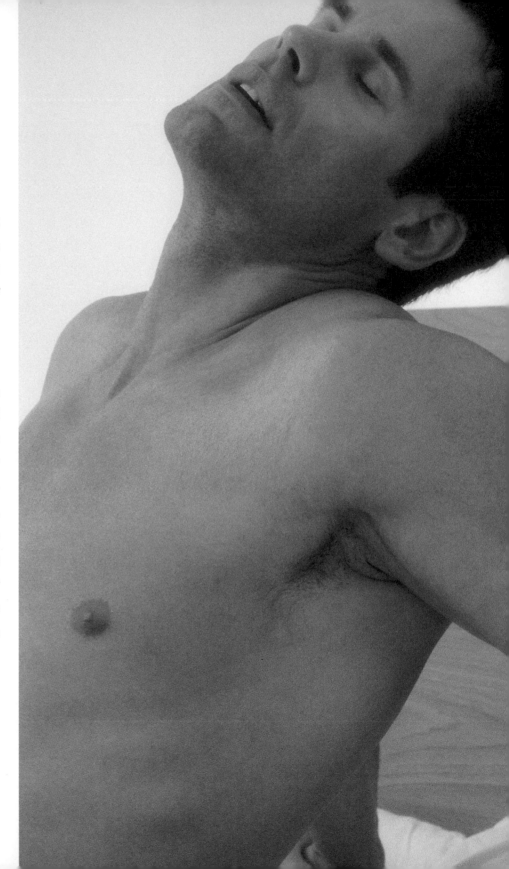

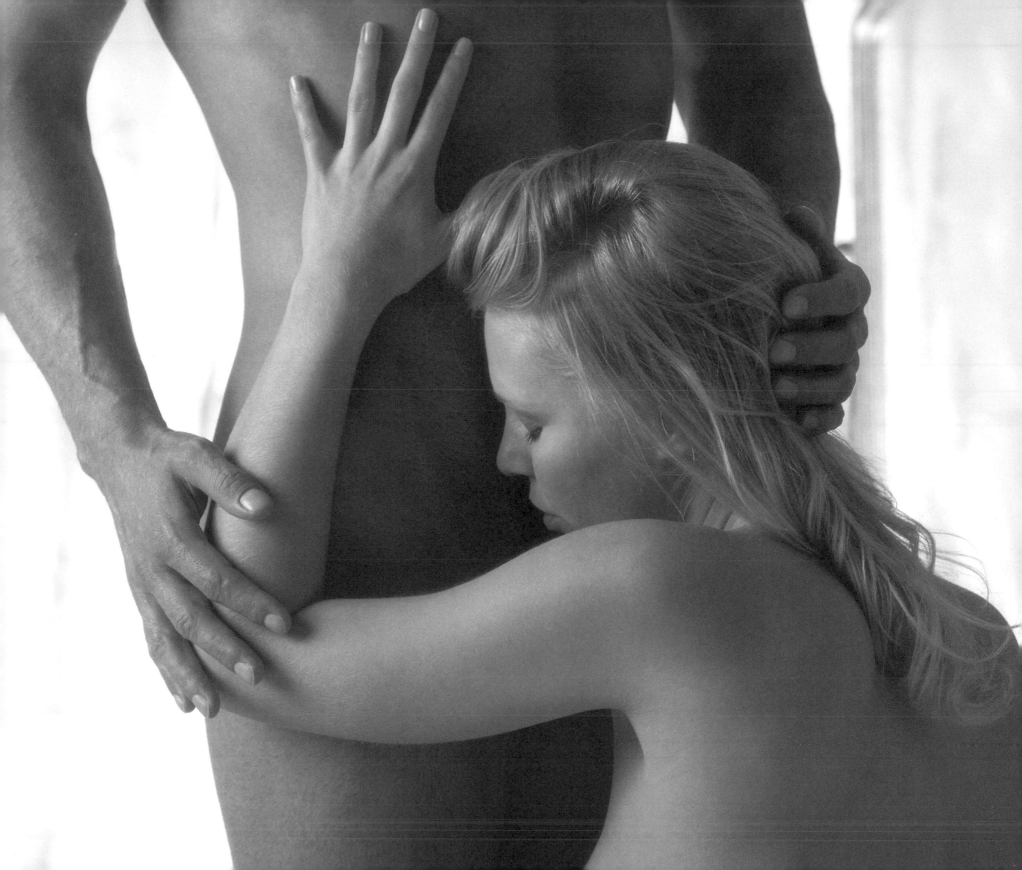

SACRED SPOTS

Imagine sex in which you stay at the peak of arousal for hours, or give yourself and your partner orgasms in which waves of pleasure ripple not just through your penis or vagina but throughout your whole body. This is achievable if you slow down your approach to sex and explore two intensely erotic zones: the Goddess Spot in women and the Sacred Spot in men.

THE GODDESS SPOT

The Goddess Spot is known by contemporary sexologists as the Grafenberg Spot – or the G-spot – after Ernst Grafenberg, the German gynecologist, who first brought this erogenous zone to public attention in the West. Although the role – and even the existence of the G-spot – has been hotly debated, the general consensus is that an area of erectile tissue inside the vagina does exist and that some women even ejaculate fluid when they reach orgasm through G-spot stimulation.

Women can find the G-spot by stroking and massaging the front wall of their vagina. Pick a time when you're feeling aroused, squat down with your knees far apart and insert your longest finger into your vagina. Apply pressure about 5cm (2 inches) up on the front wall (you may feel a swelling or lump around the size and shape of a bean or pea). Gradually increase the pressure. At first this may bring on the urge to pee. But if you keep going, this feeling can transform itself into a deep sense of erotic pleasure emanating from the core of your vagina.

If it's difficult to angle your hand in exactly the right way, try using a vibrator – you can buy one with a specially designed G-spot attachment. Alternatively, lie on your back and get your lover to stimulate your G-spot by inserting his longest finger into your vagina and then bending it into a "come-here" position.

It takes time to learn to stimulate the G-spot, especially if you want to have G-spot orgasms. The key is to be patient and don't be upset if you don't get instant results. Try stimulating the G-spot before sex to increase your vaginal sensitivity. Experiment with sex positions in which the head of his penis directly hits your G-spot (see box, opposite). Or ask your lover to massage your G-spot while you stimulate your clitoris – some women experience super-charged orgasms in this way.

POSITIONS THAT HIT THE SPOT

If you enjoy having your Goddess or Sacred Spot stimulated during sex, try these positions.

The Goddess Spot: Some of the best sex positions for Goddess Spot stimulation may be those that women naturally prefer without really realizing why. Recommended positions include women-on-top and rear-entry positions. You may also find that if you lie on your back and put your legs over your lover's shoulders, this produces strong G-spot sensations. Try: Progressing from the Yawning Position (see page 65), the Pressed Position (see page 67) or the Second Posture (see page 106). Some women find that Drawing the Bow (see page 115) is a good way to experiment with G-spot sensations during sex – try leaning further forward, in toward your lover's toes.

The Sacred Spot: Anal penetration is the only sure way of hitting a man's Sacred Spot directly during sex. But a woman can stimulate this spot indirectly by giving him a deep perineal massage while making love. The best position in which to do this is with him on his back and her astride him facing his feet.

THE SACRED SPOT

The anatomical structure that provides the amazingly sensual pleasures associated with the Sacred Spot is the prostate gland. It sits just underneath the bladder and encircles the urethra. It can be stimulated through the wall of the rectum – which is why men who have anal sex or rectal massage experience intense sensations in this area.

You can also access the Sacred Spot "remotely" by pressing deeply into the perineum. Coat your palms in massage oil, rub them together a few times and lie back on a pile of pillows with your knees spread wide apart. Put your hands between your legs and stroke firmly, applying pressure with your fingers and palms, from your anus across your perineum and up along the length of your penis. Close your eyes and concentrate on the sensations this produces. Gradually restrict your stroking to a smaller and smaller area until you are massaging a specific spot on your perineum that yields the most intense pleasure. Once you've discovered how to massage your Sacred Spot, teach your lover how to do it and start incorporating this massage into sex.

SEX STROKES

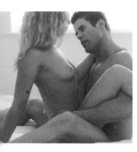

The *Kama Sutra* suggests nine different sex strokes. These are the different ways of moving the penis inside the vagina. Some of these are straightforward – for example, a technique known as "Moving Forward" describes the usual in and out movement of the penis during intercourse. Others concentrate on the angle at which the penis moves in the vagina. For example, if the head rubs one side of the vaginal wall more than the other, it is known as the "Blow of the Bull". If the penis rubs each side alternately, it is known as the "Blow of the Boar".

CHURNING AND PIERCING

Two techniques that are particularly good for clitoral stimulation during sex are Churning and Piercing. During the usual thrusting movements of intercourse, a woman's vagina receives plenty of friction but the clitoris may receive a lot less. This can make it difficult for her to reach orgasm from intercourse alone.

To try Churning: when you are both aroused, he holds his penis in his hand and she lies on her back with her legs apart. He then rubs and flicks the glans of his penis over her clitoris and

---

STROKES FOR VIGOROUS SEX

If you want forceful, vigorous sex, try the following sex strokes.

Giving a Blow: this stroke is from the *Kama Sutra*. After entering her, he withdraws completely so that the head of his penis is a short way from her vaginal entrance. Then he waits a moment and plunges into her fast and hard. He can repeat this several times during sex.

Love's Tailor: this technique is from *The Perfumed Garden*. The man puts only the head of his penis in the woman's vagina and he makes several small in and out or rubbing movements. Then, suddenly, in a single stroke, he thrusts the whole of his penis into the length of her vagina. This stroke is known as "Love's Tailor" because it is said to resemble the action of a tailor inserting his needle into a piece of fabric and then drawing it through in a single, swift pull.

Women on Top: women can also experiment with different ways of moving. For example, if she is on top, she can try fast and slow rocking, moving her hips in slow circles, or raising and lowering herself on his shaft at different speeds.

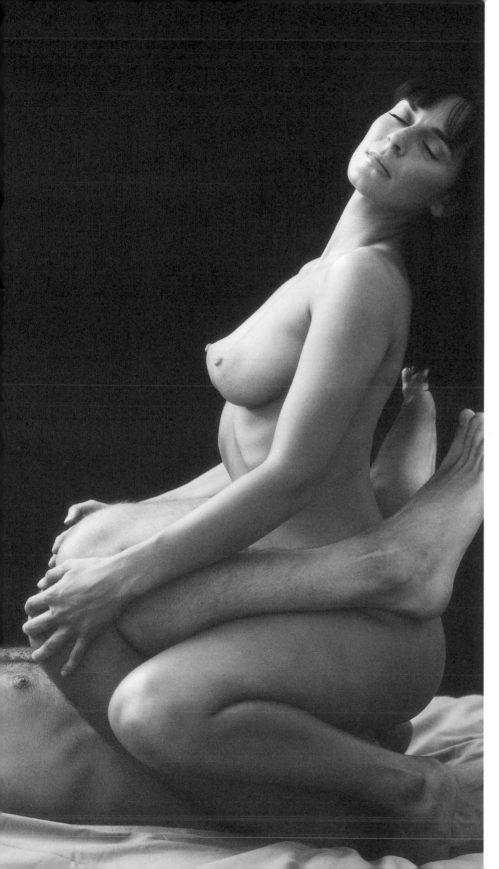

vulva until she is close to orgasm. Still holding his penis in his hand, he enters her and churns his penis in all directions.

To try Piercing: she lies down on her back and keeps her pelvis low (by not raising her hips) and he then lies high up on her body and enters her. The angle of entry is important here: rather than entering her vagina at right angles, his penis should be parallel to her vulva as he penetrates her. This means that as he moves in and out, his shaft rubs against her clitoris. (The opposite stroke to this is Rubbing, when the woman raises her pelvis and the man thrusts into her from below.)

EXPERIMENTING WITH STROKES

Make sex strokes the focus of an entire lovemaking session. Play with different ways of moving the penis inside the vagina. Discover what feels best. If you find yourselves becoming too aroused, defer climax with the *Kama Sutra* technique of Pressing: he penetrates her as deeply as possible and you both stay still in this closely joined position. When you want to come, try "Sporting of a Sparrow": he makes rapid, light, in and out strokes.

SEXUAL FIT

The way in which a couple "fit together" during sex is taken very seriously in the *Kama Sutra*. Men and women are divided into three classes depending on the length of his *lingam* and the size of her *yoni*. Today we tend not to link genital size with sexual compatibility. However, being aware of sexual fit means that you can choose the sex positions and practices that will bring you and your lover the most pleasure.

THE THREE CLASSES

Vatsyayana considered that men and women each fall into three categories. A man may be (in ascending order of penis size): a hare, a bull or a horse. Women (again, in ascending order) may be: a deer, a mare or an elephant. Today, these categories are less likely to be so strictly defined. For example, a man with a semi-erection on one occasion might be described as a hare and, on another occasion – when he is more aroused – he could be described as a bull. Likewise, a woman who has a larger vagina after childbirth can make her vagina smaller by practising pelvic floor exercises (see page 22).

EQUAL UNION

In Vatsyayana's opinion the best sexual matches between men and women are those that he describes as "equal": a hare and a deer; a bull and a mare; and a horse and an elephant.

HIGH UNION

The next best sexual matches are those that he calls "high union". Here, the man has a large penis and the woman has a small vagina in relation to the man. Examples of high union include: the horse man and the mare woman; and the bull man and the deer woman. The highest form of union is when a man with the largest penis type (a horse) has sex with a woman with the smallest vagina type (a deer).

LOW UNION

According to Vatsyayana the least satisfying sexual match is between a man with a small penis and a woman with a comparatively large vagina. He calls this "low congress". Sex between an elephant woman and a bull man or a mare woman and a hare

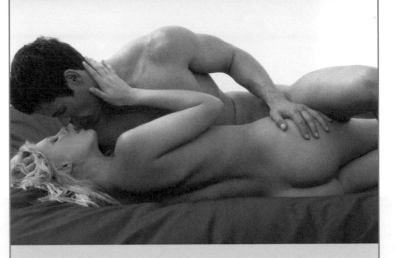

man are examples of low congress. The lowest form of congress is between the elephant woman and the hare man.

TAILORING SEX

There are several ways that you can enhance sex if the sexual fit between you is unequal. In cases of high union, you should begin intercourse only when she is fully aroused and lubricated (this is because arousal causes the upper part of the vagina to expand, making more room for the penis). You can also use an extra lubricant such as a water-soluble jelly to make penetration more comfortable. Above all, allow the woman to guide the depth of penetration and the pace of lovemaking and let her choose the sex positions that feel most comfortable.

In cases of low union, a woman can make her lover feel more tightly "held" by contracting her love muscles (see pages 22–3). If she regularly exercises these muscles, she can achieve a toned vagina that will enhance sexual sensation for both of you. Some couples also find that it helps to insert fingers or a small vibrator alongside the penis during intercourse.

SEX POSITIONS TO MAXIMIZE SENSATION

High Union: choose woman-on-top positions such as the Contrary Position (see page 85) or the Large Bee (see page 89). These let her guide his penis into her slowly, and control the movements of lovemaking. Man-on-top or side-by-side positions in which the penis doesn't deeply penetrate the vagina are also good: try the Supine Clasping Position (see page 56), the Side-by-side Clasping Position (see page 57), the Lotus Position (see page 74) or the Transverse Position (see page 80).

Low Union: choose man-on-top sex positions in which the penis penetrates the vagina as deeply as possible, such as the Position of Indrani (see page 66) or the Pressed Position (see page 67). Rear-entry positions are also good; try Congress of a Cow (see page 63), the Elephant Pose (see page 88) or the Ninth Posture (see page 104).

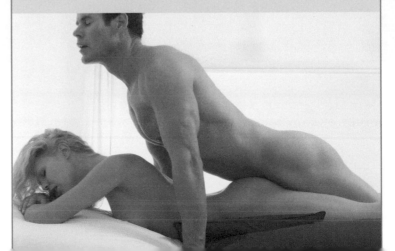

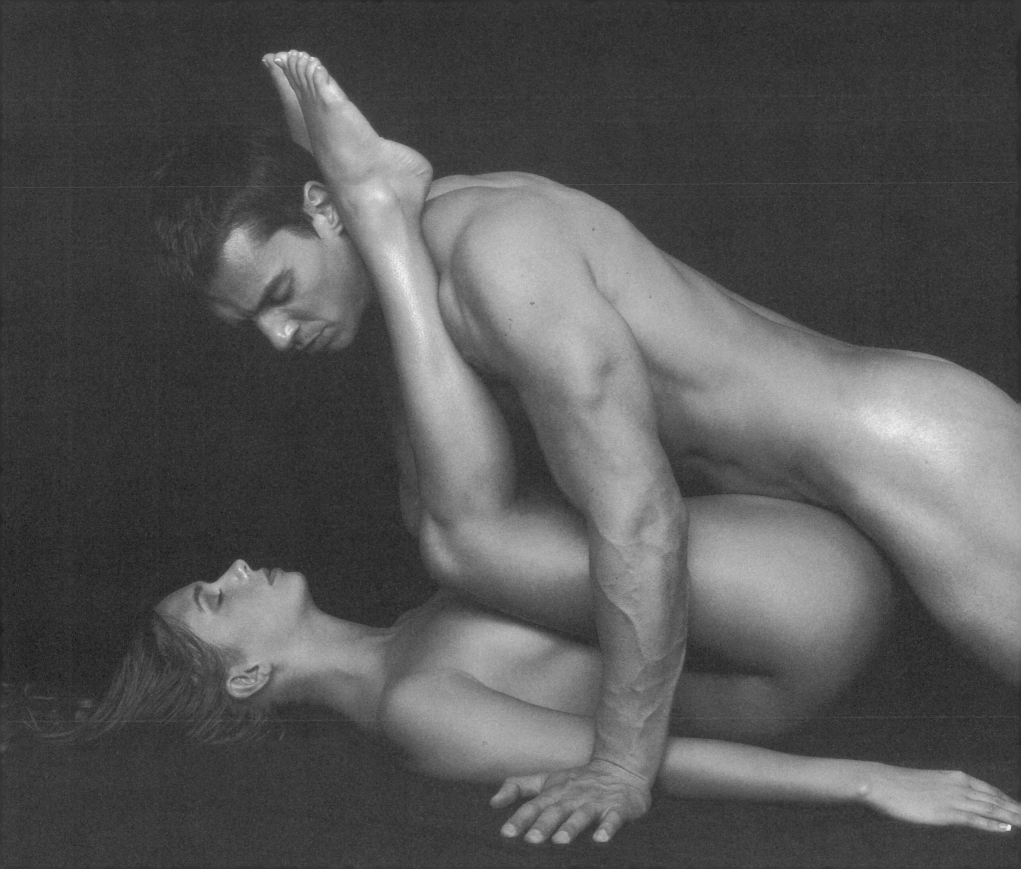

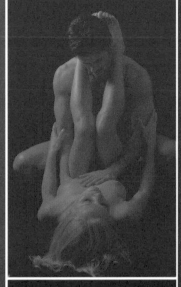

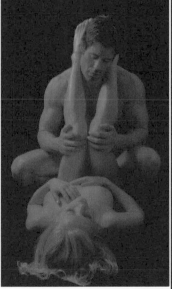

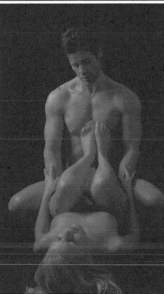

CHAPTER 3

RIDING THE
WAVE OF E

KAMA SUTRA • ANANGA RANGA • TH

KAMA SUTRA POSITIONS

If you enjoy man-on-top positions there are plenty in the *Kama Sutra*. The majority of sex positions described by Vatsyayana consist of the woman lying on her back with her legs at a variety of angles from relaxed on the bed to folded into the tightly-packed yoga position, the lotus. Great things about man-on-top positions include the pressure of the man's pubic bone on the clitoris, the potential for deep penetration, the intimacy of being face-to-face and the eroticism of female surrender and male dominance. Because many of the positions are similar – sometimes there are only small differences in the angle of the woman's legs – your challenge as lovers is to discover the stimulation produced by these small position changes. As experienced yogis can testify (many of the *Kama Sutra* positions are derived from Hatha yoga), sometimes it takes just a tiny change, such as a slight shift in the angle of a limb, to have a dramatically different effect on the rest of the body. Rather than thrusting vigorously in the following sex positions, take the time to lie still and quietly together and observe the different sensations produced by the woman raising or lowering her legs or moving her knees closer or further away from her chest or the sides of her body.

In addition to the positions described on the following pages, Vatsyayana describes two embraces that can be used at the time of sexual union. The first, the "Mixture of Sesamum Seed With Rice", describes how two lovers lying down on a bed can encircle each other with their arms and legs. In the second, the "Milk and Water Embrace", the woman sits on the man's lap and the couple embrace each other as if they were entering each other's body "without any thought of pain or hurt".

SLOW AND SOULFUL

These six *Kama Sutra* positions are designed for sex that's really up-close-and-personal. You can whisper to each other and exchange licks, bites and passionate kisses that make you feel truly connected both in mind and body. Because the positions are face-to-face you can also enjoy the intoxicating experience of observing each other's expressions during sex. These positions enable affectionate, intimate lovemaking for when you want to really get inside each other's skin. If you like lots of position changes during sex, you can do most of these positions one after the other.

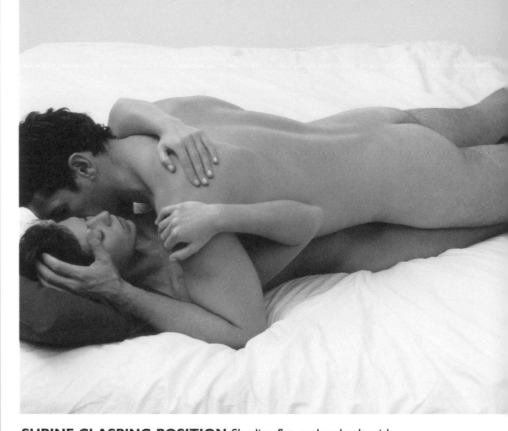

SUPINE CLASPING POSITION She lies flat on her back with her legs apart and he climbs on top and enters her. Both of you have your legs stretched out straight. This is a wonderful position in which to lie still at the beginning or end of sex and just savour the feeling of being so intimately joined. Lying together like this at the beginning of sex really builds up sexual tension — the urge for him to thrust will soon feel irresistible! Use this position to gaze deeply into each other's eyes or exchange a long, passionate kiss. She can also try contracting her vaginal muscles around his penis in this position.

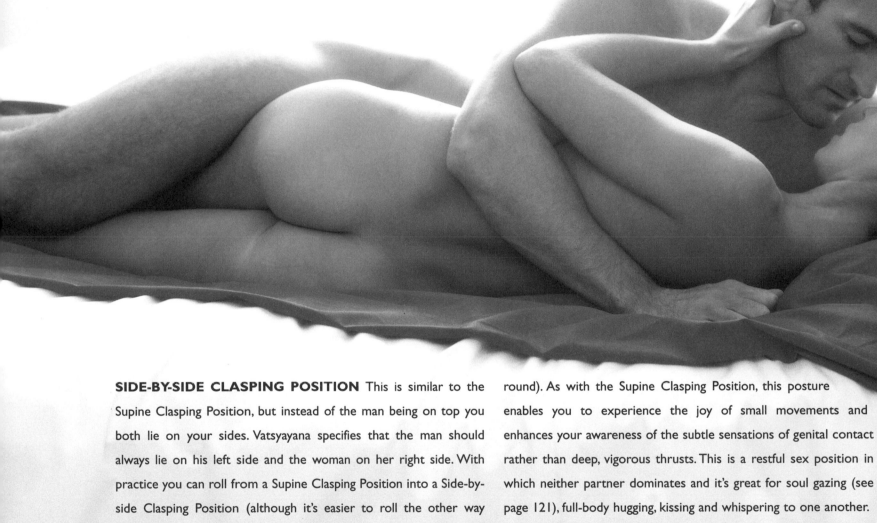

SIDE-BY-SIDE CLASPING POSITION This is similar to the Supine Clasping Position, but instead of the man being on top you both lie on your sides. Vatsyayana specifies that the man should always lie on his left side and the woman on her right side. With practice you can roll from a Supine Clasping Position into a Side-by-side Clasping Position (although it's easier to roll the other way round). As with the Supine Clasping Position, this posture enables you to experience the joy of small movements and enhances your awareness of the subtle sensations of genital contact rather than deep, vigorous thrusts. This is a restful sex position in which neither partner dominates and it's great for soul gazing (see page 121), full-body hugging, kissing and whispering to one another.

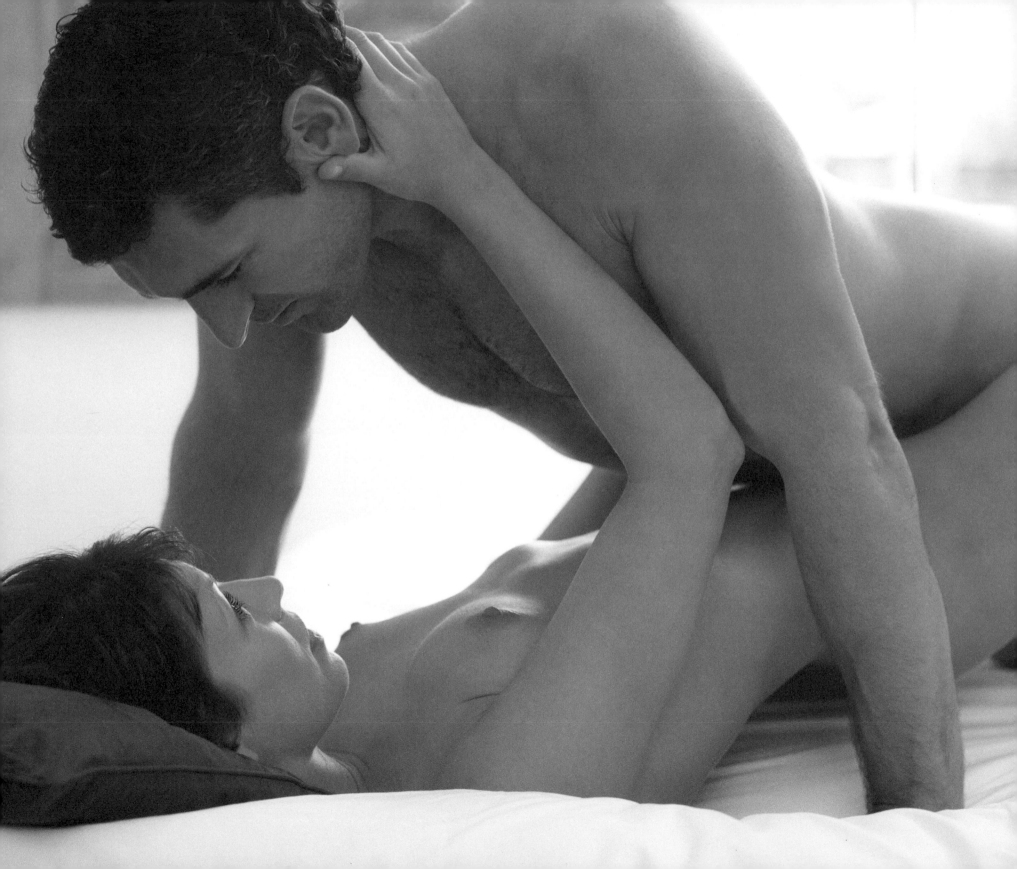

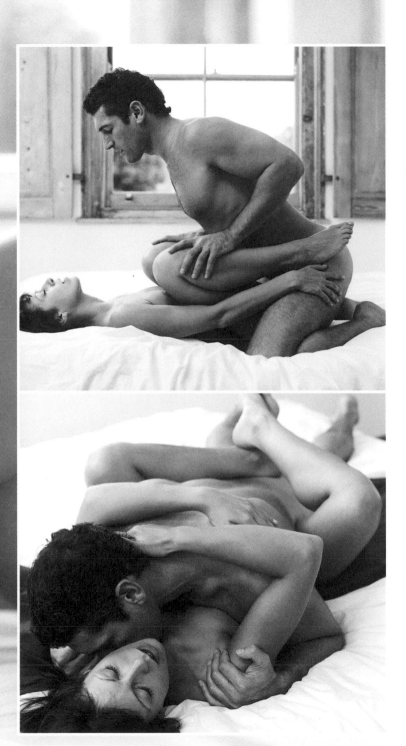

WIDELY-OPENED POSITION (main image) He lies on top and penetrates her. She then bends her knees, puts her feet flat on the bed and raises her pelvis. He can thrust inside her or remain still while she moves her pelvis up and down. Even if she can't hold this position for very long it's a sexy "in-between" position that allows the man to feel the eroticism of her body rising up to meet his.

CRAB'S POSITION (inset, top) She lies on her back, bends her knees and draws her thighs toward her stomach. He lies or kneels between her legs and enters her. If he holds her knees firmly she can relax her legs and feel a powerful sense of letting go in this position.

PRESSING POSITION (inset, bottom) Begin in a Supine Clasping Position (see page 56), then she bends her legs and presses his body with her thighs. She can do this with her feet flat on the bed or with her thighs raised. To create a compelling sense of intimacy and being quite literally wrapped up in one another, she can rest her calves on his lower back and cross her ankles.

TWINING POSITION He lies on top of her and after penetration she raises one leg and wraps it around the back of his thigh (you can also make love in this position when you are standing up; see Supported Congress on page 63). Raising her leg in this way gives the woman more control over lovemaking: she can use pressure from her leg to push him in and out, which means that she guides the rhythm and pace of penetration. If she is strong and supple enough, she can use the heel of her foot to massage his buttocks or to apply pressure to his perineum (the area between the anus and the genitals) – touching this area can lead to swift and powerful orgasms in some men. To increase or decrease the depth of his penis in her vagina she can move her leg higher up or lower down his body.

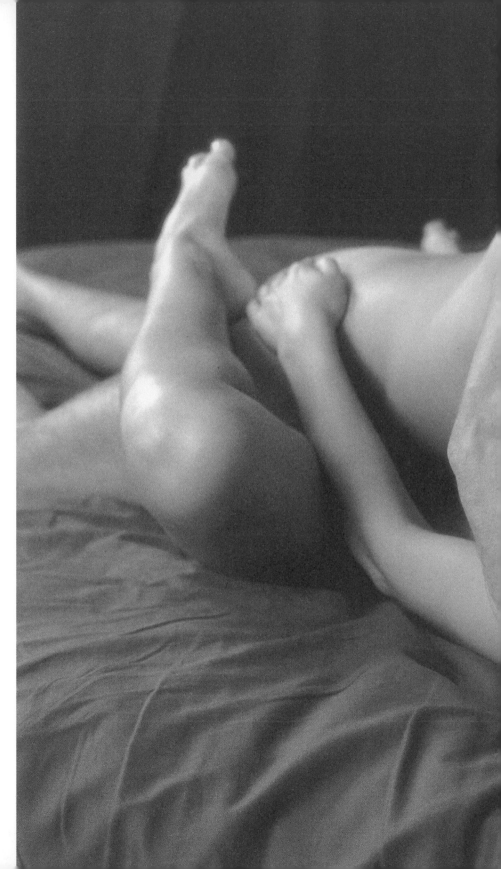

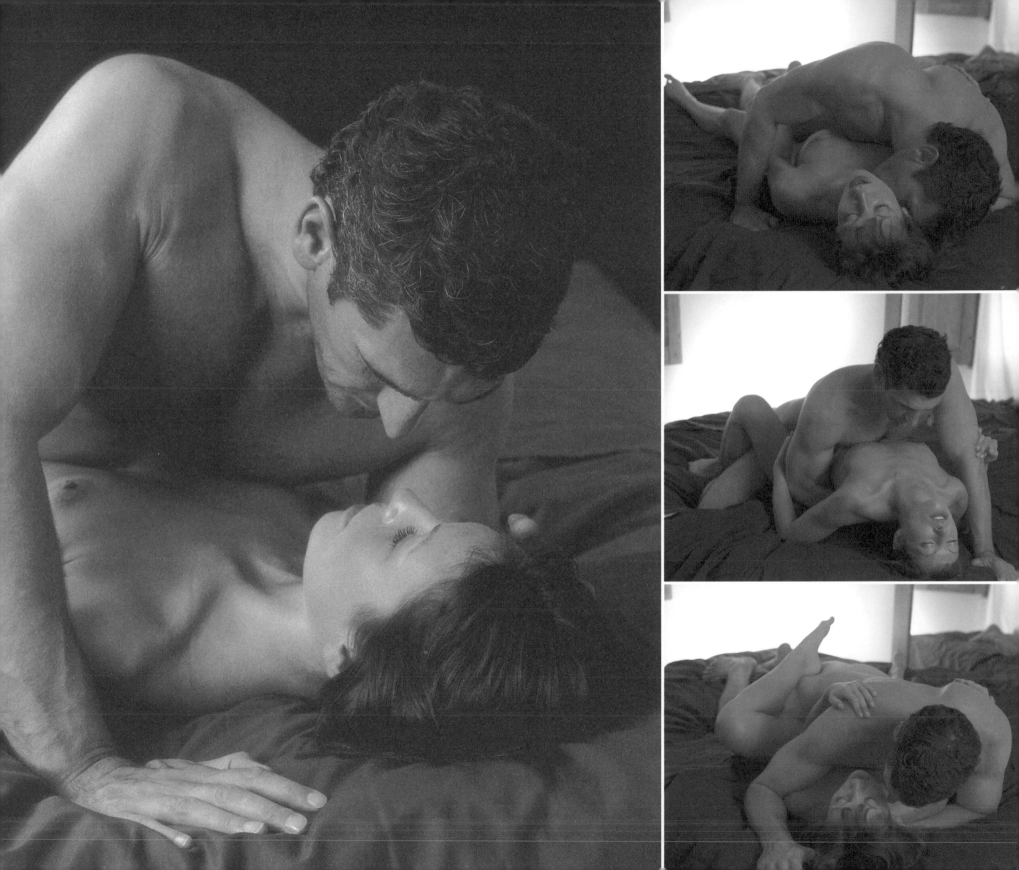

FAST AND PASSIONATE

Some of the most exciting and memorable sex happens

spontaneously in a place where you wouldn't normally think

of having sex. These three positions from the *Kama Sutra* lend

themselves to impromptu sex when you don't have much

time and there is no bed or convenient surface on which to

lie down. Supported Congress and Congress of a Cow are

best suited to couples who are roughly the same height.

Suspended Congress is a great position for women who are

small and light, although a heavier woman can take a fair bit

of her own weight by pressing her feet against the wall.

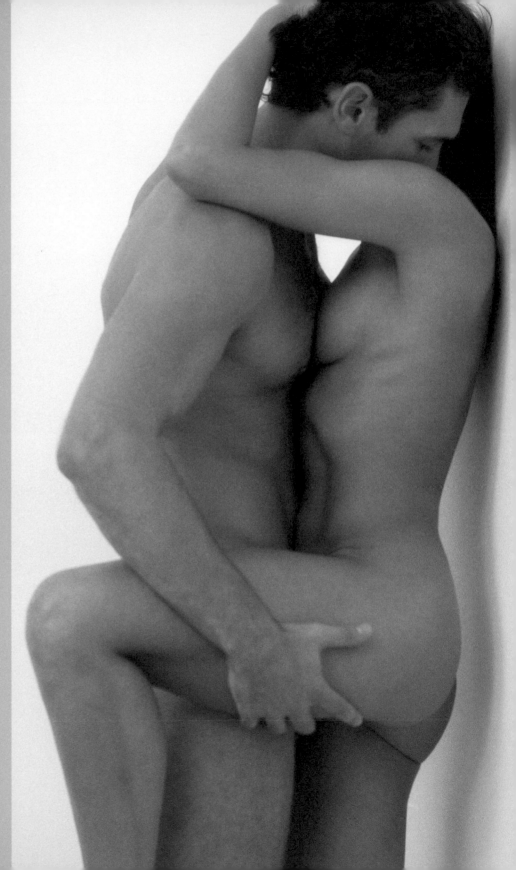

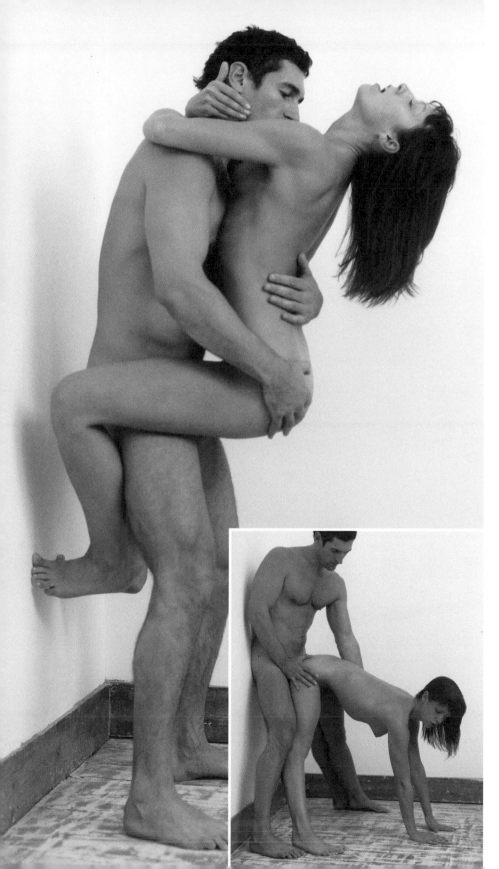

SUPPORTED CONGRESS (far left) This is a classic quickie position – you don't even have to get completely undressed. She stands with her back against a wall while he presses his body to hers. She wraps one leg around him – the higher her leg the better – and he enters her. If you enjoy having sex in the shower, try this position.

SUSPENDED CONGRESS (left) This position in which he stands against a wall, lifts her and clasps his hands underneath her buttocks is perfect for fast sex when you're both at the peak of arousal. She moves up and down on his penis by pushing against the wall with her feet. If you can't do this for long, he can kneel down and you can move seamlessly into the Pressing Position (see page 59).

CONGRESS OF A COW (inset) She bends over so that her hands touch the floor and the man enters her from behind. This animalistic position evokes powerful and erotic feelings of dominance and vulnerability in men and women. The anonymity of this position – in that you can't see each other's faces – can be a huge turn-on. Feel free to indulge your wildest sexual fantasies.

DEEP AND EROTIC

These seven positions from the *Kama Sutra* offer ways for the

man to enter the woman very deeply. This is because, with the

exception of the Mare's Position, the woman's legs are either

at right angles to her body or one or both of her knees are

drawn toward her chest – this has the effect of contracting

the vagina. If you find deep penetration uncomfortable, stick

with the Yawning Position in which the woman's legs form

a natural barrier and prevent the fullest possible penetration.

If, on the other hand, you enjoy deep penetration, go straight

into the Position of Indrani or the Pressed Position.

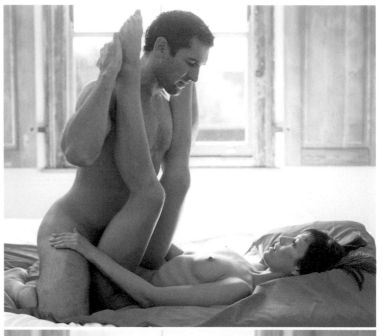

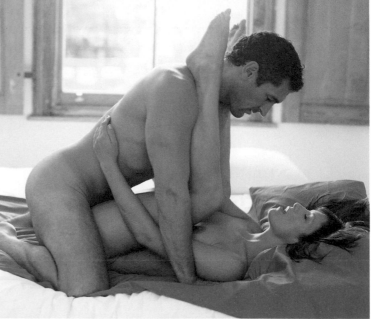

YAWNING POSITION (left, top) She lies on her back and raises her legs to rest along the front of his body. He can hold her hands for support as he thrusts. In a variation of this position he can hold onto her feet and gently push them apart (see illustration), this will give him the sensation that she is opening up to him – she needs to be fairly supple in the groin for this position.

PROGRESSING FROM THE YAWNING POSITION (left, bottom) She brings her knees to her shoulders and rests her feet on his shoulders. He should start by thrusting slowly and gently. She can give him feedback.

MARE'S POSITION Strictly speaking, this is a technique rather than a position. After penetration, the woman tightly contracts her love muscles (see pages 22–3) so that the man feels tightly held – this takes practice. You can try this technique in any sex position, but it works especially well when the woman sits on the man's lap facing away from him (see illustration, right). Once you've perfected the vaginal squeeze, try a pumping and a fluttering action.

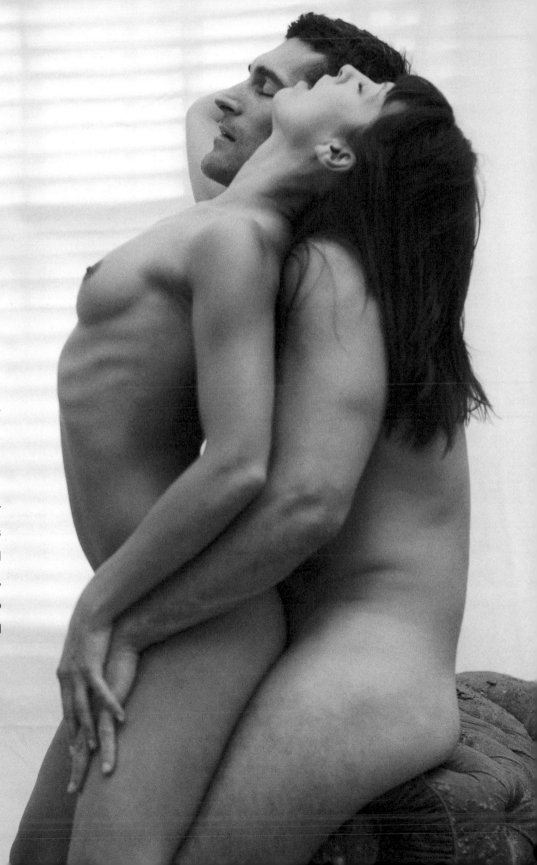

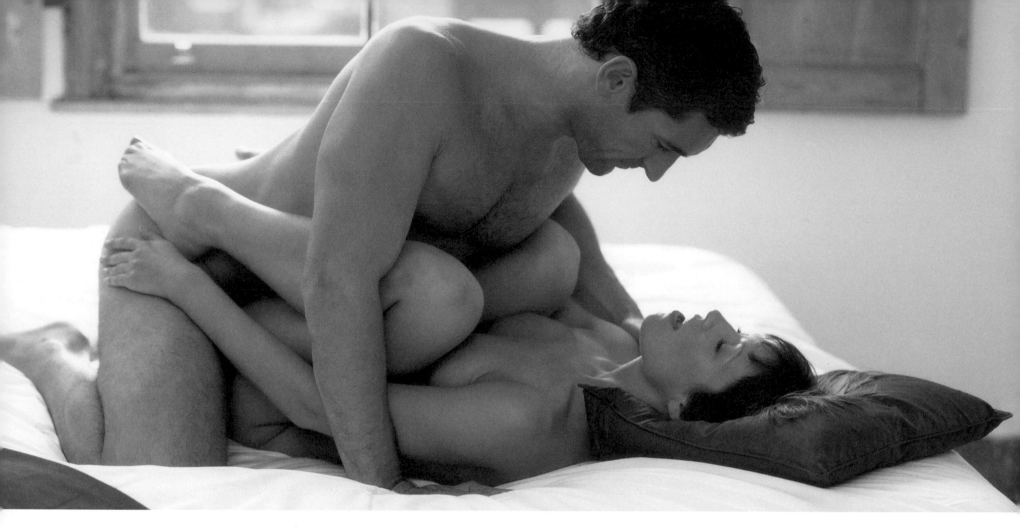

POSITION OF INDRANI This position, in which the woman draws her knees up to the sides of her body, is recommended in the *Kama Sutra* for the hare man (with a short penis) because it enables the woman to feel deeply penetrated. The elephant man (with a large penis) should take care in this position because penetration can be uncomfortable or even painful if the penis hits the cervix – it's best to go slowly and wait until the woman is extremely aroused (the upper vagina expands and the uterus lifts at the peak of sexual excitement and this creates more space for the penis). You may not be able to have fast and furious sex in this position, but lots of couples rate it as one of the best in terms of intensity and eroticism. Try communicating with your eyes alone.

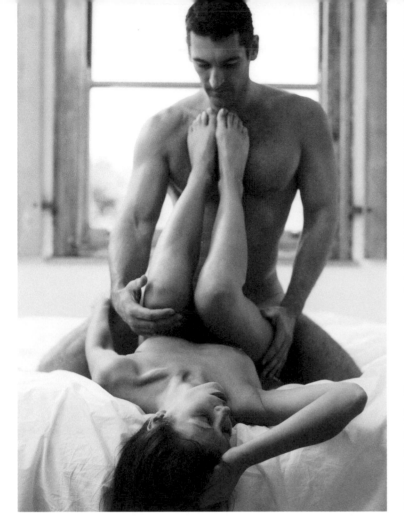
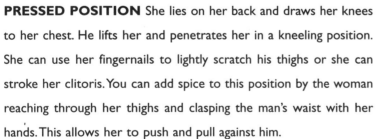
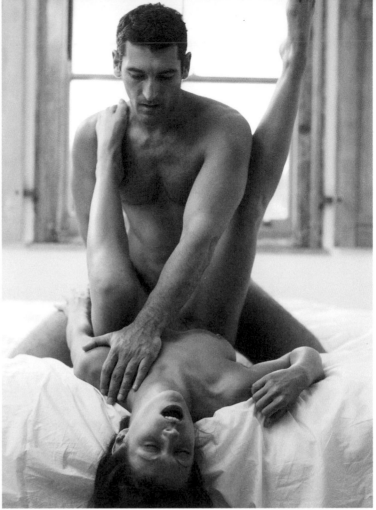

PRESSED POSITION She lies on her back and draws her knees to her chest. He lifts her and penetrates her in a kneeling position. She can use her fingernails to lightly scratch his thighs or she can stroke her clitoris. You can add spice to this position by the woman reaching through her thighs and clasping the man's waist with her hands. This allows her to push and pull against him.

HALF-PRESSED POSITION After the Pressed Position she stretches out one of her legs so that her foot points to the ceiling. This changes the sensations she experiences by creating more space in the vagina, and provides a break from the intensity of extremely deep penetration. It's also easier for the woman to stroke her clitoris in this position.

RISING POSITION She lies on her back with her legs raised in the air to make a wide "V" shape (she should spread her legs as far apart as she can) and he leans between her legs to enter her. An advantage of the Rising Position for the man is that he can lean back and watch his penis moving in and out of her vagina. If the depth of the penis feels too intense in this position, she can bend her knees and put her feet on the bed. If she wants to be penetrated more deeply, she can draw her knees to her chest. Experiment with the angle of her legs to find out what feels best for both of you.

ADVENTUROUS

The majority of these five *Kama Sutra* positions present a challenge to the woman in that she needs to be flexible in her hips and groin to be able to lift and support her legs in a variety of poses. The Lotus Position demands that she be able to do some fairly advanced yoga (but don't worry – there's an easier alternative!). An adventurous position for men is the Turning Position. This requires considerable skill and dexterity as he starts in a man-on-top position and then attempts to complete a 180-degree body turn while remaining inside his lover.

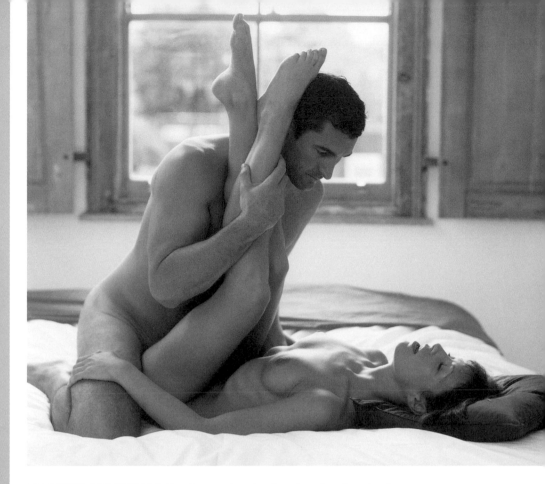

PACKED POSITION She lies on her back, raises her legs in the air and crosses them. She can either rest her crossed legs on one of his shoulders after he has entered her or he can treat her legs as a vertical pole to hold on to. The woman has little freedom to move in this position, which may mean that you want to maintain it for only a short time. Alternatively, the element of female surrender and male dominance can be arousing for both of you.

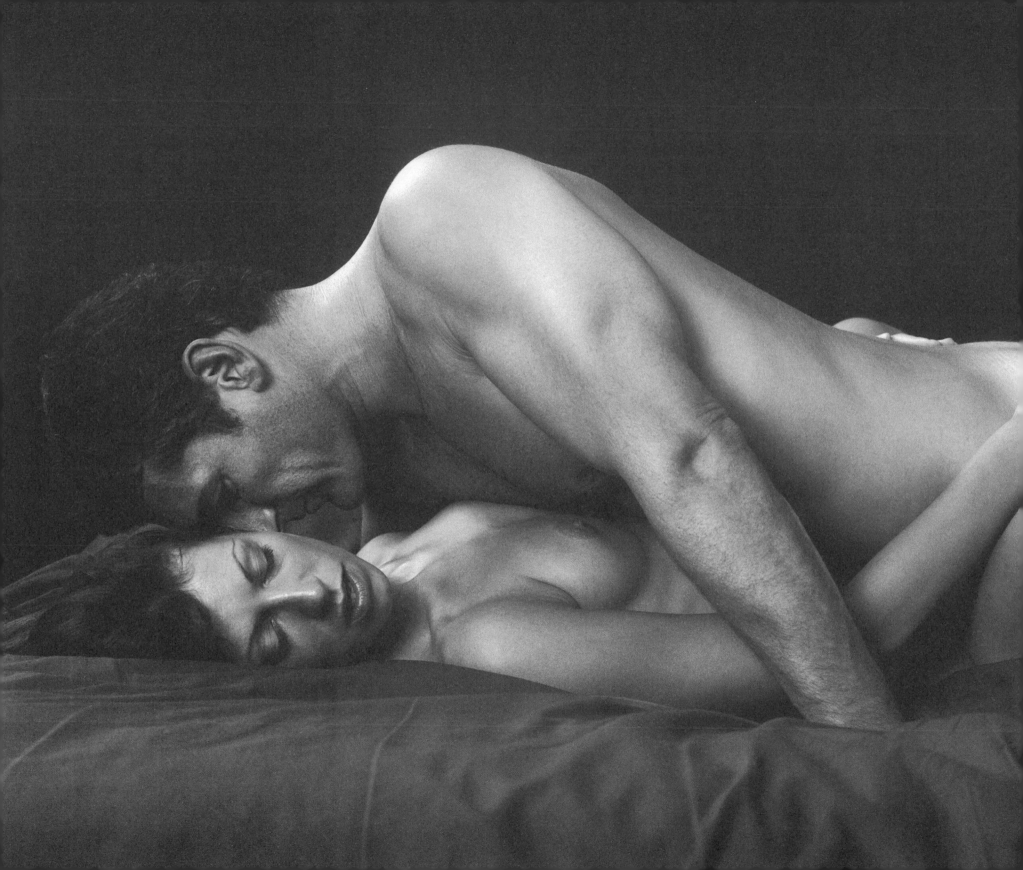

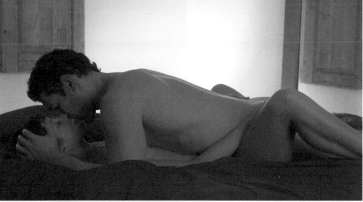

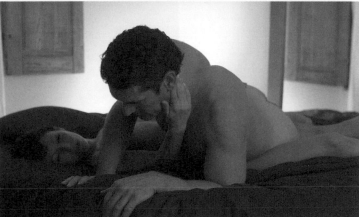

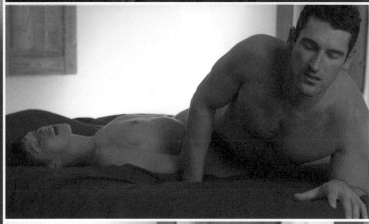

TURNING POSITION This is a challenging but fun position that is really four positions in one. As the man turns around, his penis moves in the women's vagina by 180 degrees – this creates new sensations for both of you.

1. Start in a man-on-top position with his legs between hers. Wait for a time when you're ready for a change of position – he needs to have a strong erection but not be on the verge of ejaculating.

2. He pushes himself up on his hands and withdraws slightly to give himself room to maneuver. Then he moves his right leg so that it rests on the outside of her left leg. His pelvis should still be pressed close to hers.

3. He brings his left leg to join his right one and moves his body so that he lies over her to form a cross-shape. Because he is still inside her, he can thrust a few times to maintain his erection.

4. He carefully completes the turn so that his penis doesn't slip out of her. Now he can gently move his hips from side to side in this position while she kneads or scratches his buttocks. This is also a great position if you both love toe-sucking!

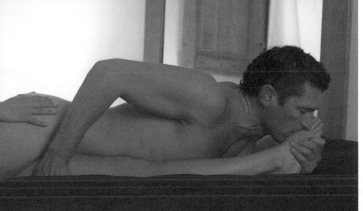

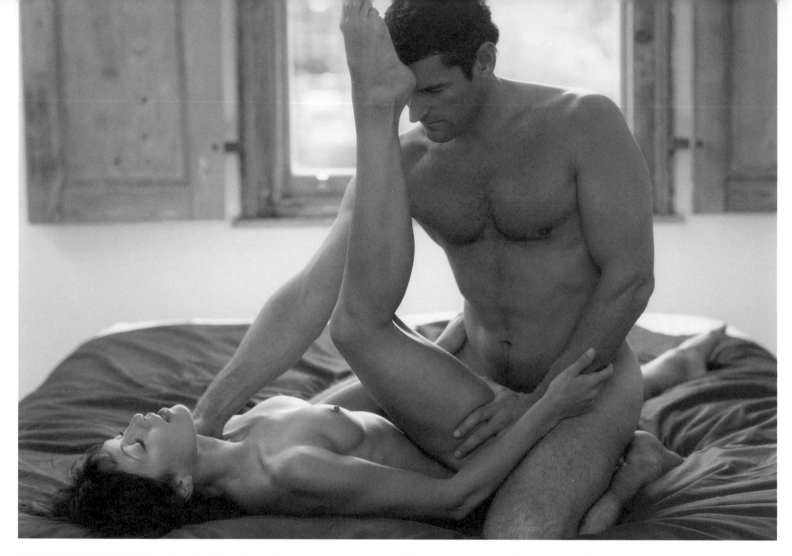

FIXING OF A NAIL In this playful position she stretches one leg out on the floor or bed and rests the heel of her other foot on his forehead. Her raised foot acts as a hammer that knocks the nail – his head! – into a wall. For her to keep her heel on his forehead love-making needs to be slow and considered rather than fast and furious.

You can even try lying perfectly still in this position while she contracts her love muscles around his penis (see page 23). Meanwhile, he can move her foot down to his mouth and cover the sole in kisses before sucking each one of her toes. You can move seamlessly from this position into the next: Splitting of a Bamboo.

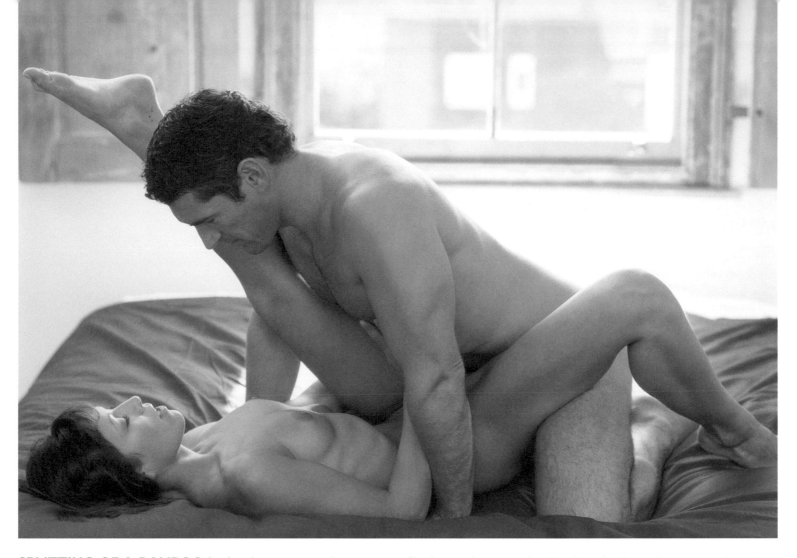

SPLITTING OF A BAMBOO In this dynamic pose the woman changes the positions of her legs throughout lovemaking. She starts with one leg hooked over the man's shoulder and one leg stretched out on the floor or bed. Then she moves the upright leg down and the stretched leg up (he can help her lift her legs up and down). She keeps alternating her legs like this for as long as you both hold the position. The main benefit of this is that the angle of the penis in the vagina keeps changing, producing a variety of sensations for both of you. Depending on the suppleness of the woman, the man can lie on top and kiss her mouth or kneel in an upright position.

LOTUS POSITION The Lotus is an advanced yoga pose that you should practise by yourself before you attempt it during sex: sit on the floor or bed in an upright position. Bend your right leg and tuck your right heel tightly into your left hip socket. Now lift your left foot up onto your right thigh as close to your right hip socket as you can. Even sustaining this yoga pose for a short time on a regular basis will have a beneficial effect on the flexibility of your hips and groin. If you find this pose easy, try getting into it while lying down – now let your lover enter you. Some women enjoy the tight, compact nature of this position during sex, but it may be hard to maintain. If you find the Lotus Position difficult or uncomfortable, just cross your legs instead.

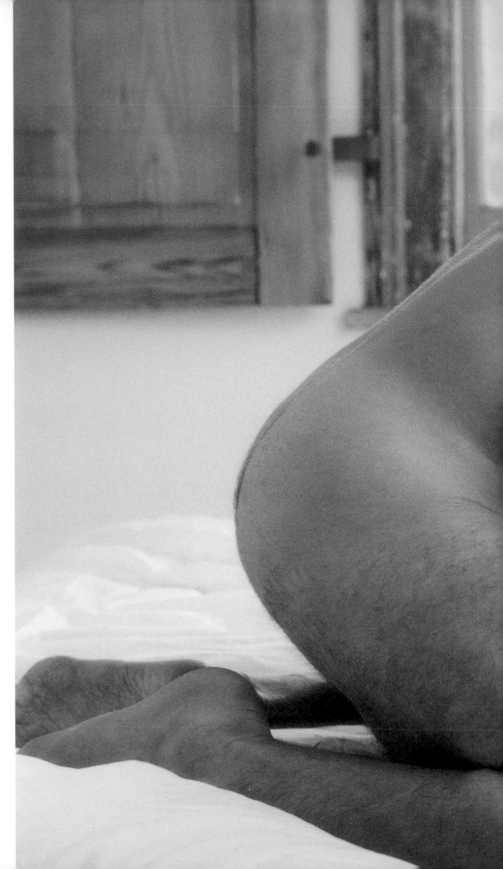

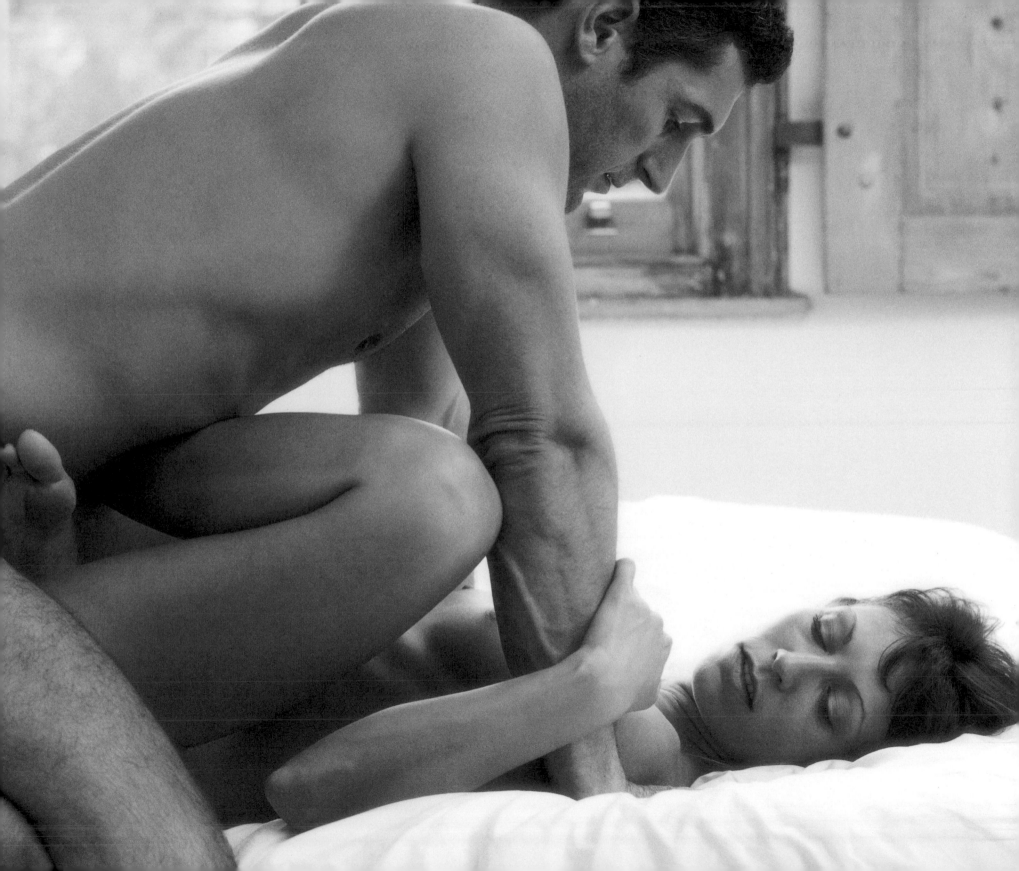

KAMA SUTRA SEQUENCE

If you love multiple-position sex, this sequence should challenge even the most athletic of

lovers. Begin with some raunchy standing-up sex in Supported Congress and Suspended

Congress. Try to stay connected as you move into a lying down position – it's tricky but

possible. Now move through the five face-to-face man-on-top positions shown in the

pictures: you begin in a Pressing Position and progress through three positions in which

her legs are raised at varying angles, then she brings her legs down onto the bed and you

finish in the Supine Clasping position. He may need to withdraw before you get into the

two final positions, but once you're sitting in the Mare's Position you can both stand up

and move seamlessly into Congress of a Cow.

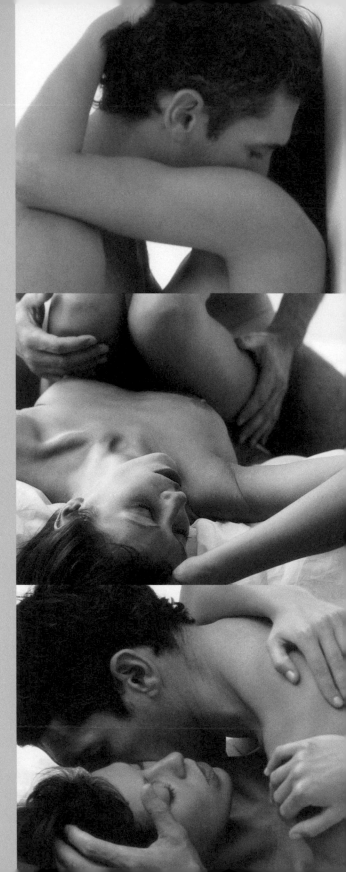

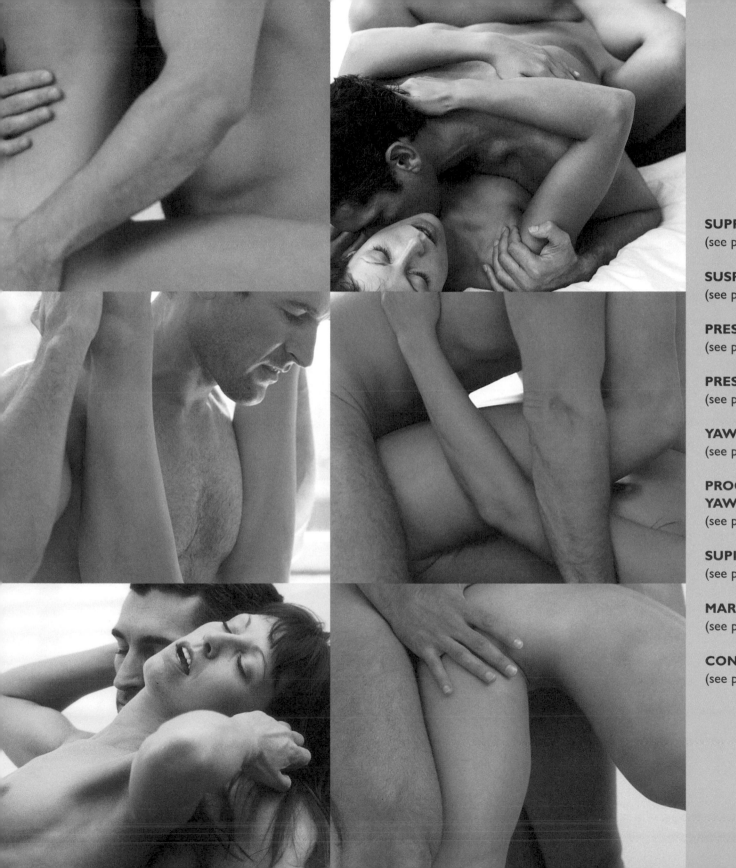

ANANGA RANGA POSITIONS

Kalyana Malla, the author of the *Ananga Ranga*, recommends that before lovers have sex, they indulge in "external enjoyments", such as kisses, caresses or embraces. These, he says, serve to divert the mind from coyness and coldness and excite the passions of both partners. In particular they arouse the woman and loosen her *yoni* (see page 18) in preparation for sex. Malla believes in the premise that a rich and varied sex life will compel couples to stay together. To this end he presents 32 different sex positions (a selection of the most erotic are shown on the following pages) so that lovers may enjoy each other as if they had 32 different partners.

As well as presenting a selection of standing and lying poses, the *Ananga Ranga* suggests a range of sitting positions in which to make love. The advantages of these positions are that neither partner dominates, the woman can touch her clitoris freely (either with her hand or with a vibrator), and you can gaze into your lover's eyes and kiss. If you are practising Tantric sex (see Chapter 4) and are concentrating on breathing and harnessing sexual energy, sitting positions are ideal.

The *Ananga Ranga* suggests three woman-on-top sex positions. In each one it is recommended that the woman squeezes her love muscles (see pages 22–3) in the same way that a hand opens and closes to milk a cow. Malla advises that although this takes much practice and an intense focus on the muscles concerned, the benefits will be great. As well as intensifying her own experience of sex, the woman will ensure that her partner will never exchange her – not even for the most beautiful queen!

SLOW AND SOULFUL

These six positions from the *Ananga Ranga* offer a variety of ways to enjoy sex that is gentle and unhurried, from the intimately entwined Thigh Clasp to the expansive "spread out" nature of the Foot Clasp. Most of these positions aren't suitable for free and vigorous thrusting, but they are perfect for nurturing a sense of connection and for savouring the subtler sensations of being penetrated and enclosed. The Bow Position is one of the few positions for which you require props – make sure you have a pile of cushions or pillows to hand before you begin.

THIGH CLASP He lies on his side between her thighs (she wraps one thigh over him and one thigh underneath him). He will feel tightly enclosed, but neither partner is dominant in this position. It's fairly easy for her to reach between her legs to stroke her clitoris, he can caress her breasts and there is the opportunity for lots of eye contact and kissing. There are also plenty of ways to vary or extend this position, so explore it and find out what you and your partner most enjoy. For example, both partners can move their bodies apart to form a wide "V" shape. Or she can try rolling onto her back and hooking both of her legs over his upper hip.

TRANSVERSE POSITION (inset) The man lies on his side, facing the woman. He raises his upper leg and puts it over her hip. Depending on the individual anatomy of you and your partner, you may find that you can achieve only shallow penetration in this position. One idea for increasing the eroticism of the Transverse Position is to use some massage oil on your belly and genitals so that you slip and slide against each other during lovemaking (but don't use oil if you are also using a condom – oil damages latex).

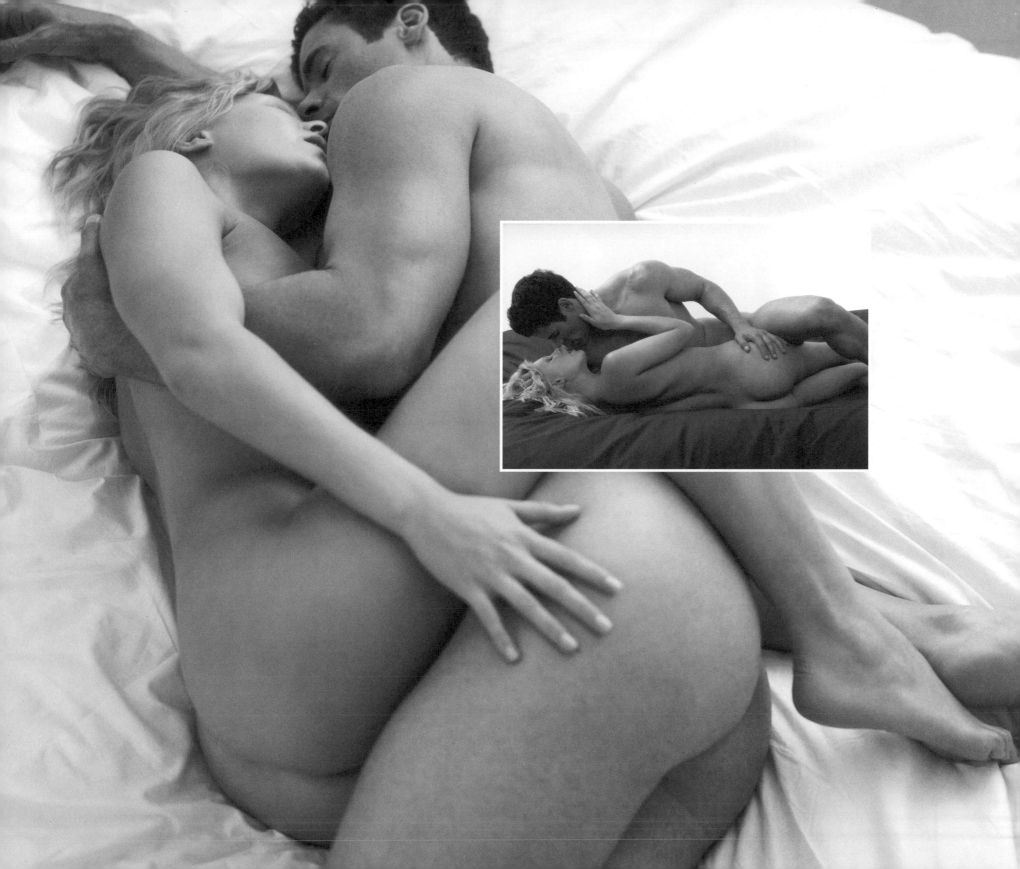

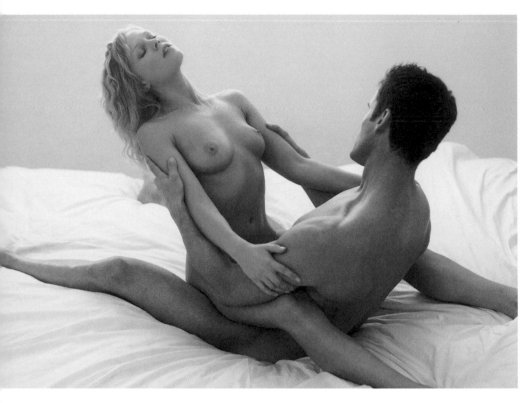

KAMA'S WHEEL He sits on the floor or a bed with his legs stretched out in front of him and she then sits astride him with her legs straight out behind his body. You both hold onto each other's upper body. This is a sexy alternative to making love lying down and you can get into it directly from a woman-on-top position. Once you've been in this position for a while the woman can lie back on the floor or the bed to expose her clitoris and, remaining inside her, the man can bring her to orgasm using his fingers or thumb.

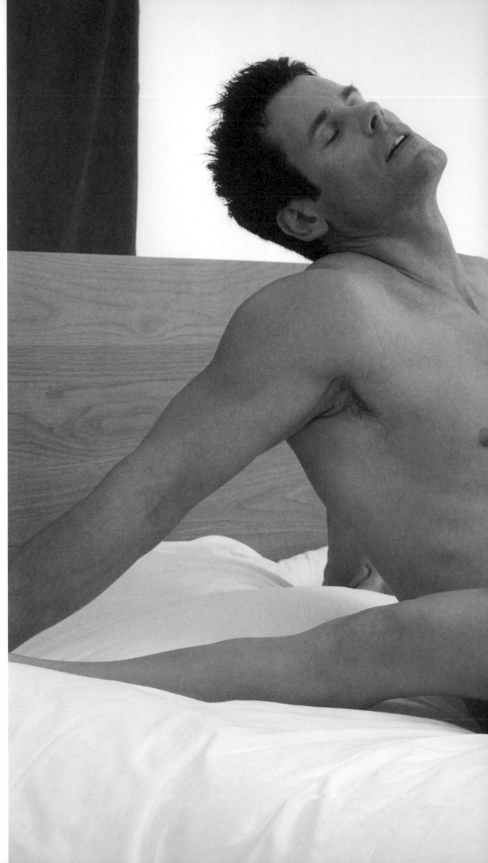

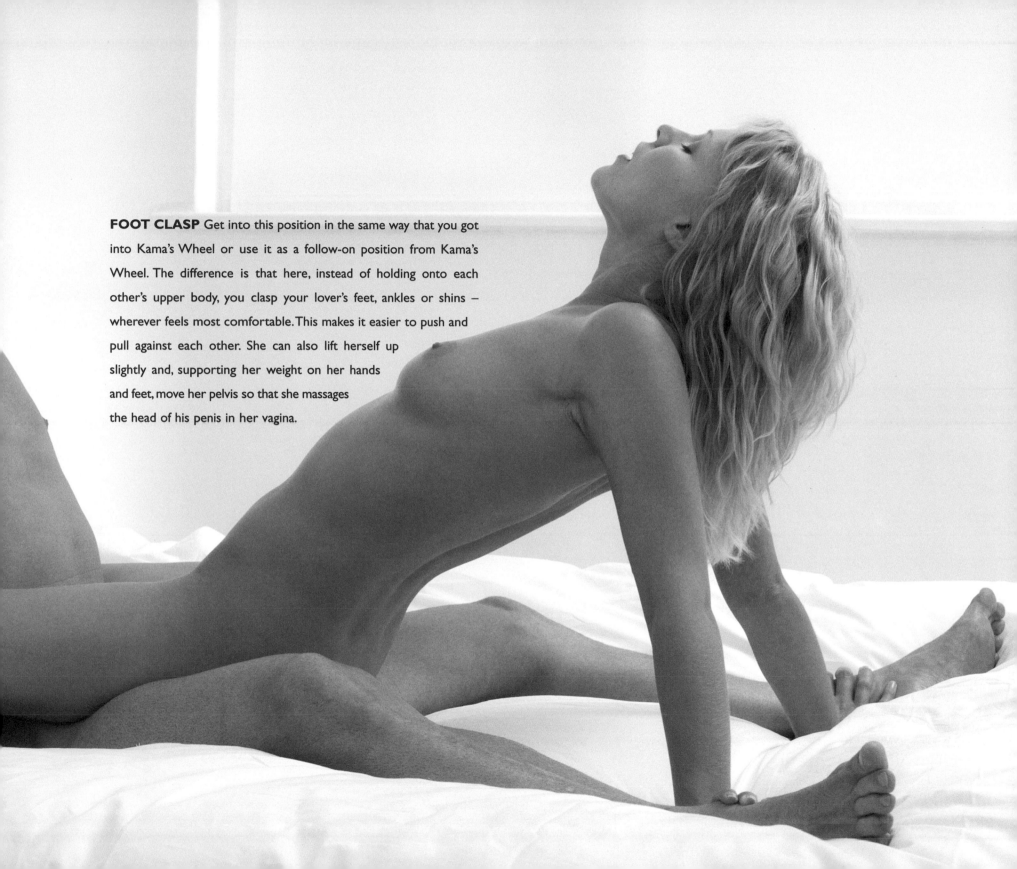

FOOT CLASP Get into this position in the same way that you got into Kama's Wheel or use it as a follow-on position from Kama's Wheel. The difference is that here, instead of holding onto each other's upper body, you clasp your lover's feet, ankles or shins — wherever feels most comfortable. This makes it easier to push and pull against each other. She can also lift herself up slightly and, supporting her weight on her hands and feet, move her pelvis so that she massages the head of his penis in her vagina.

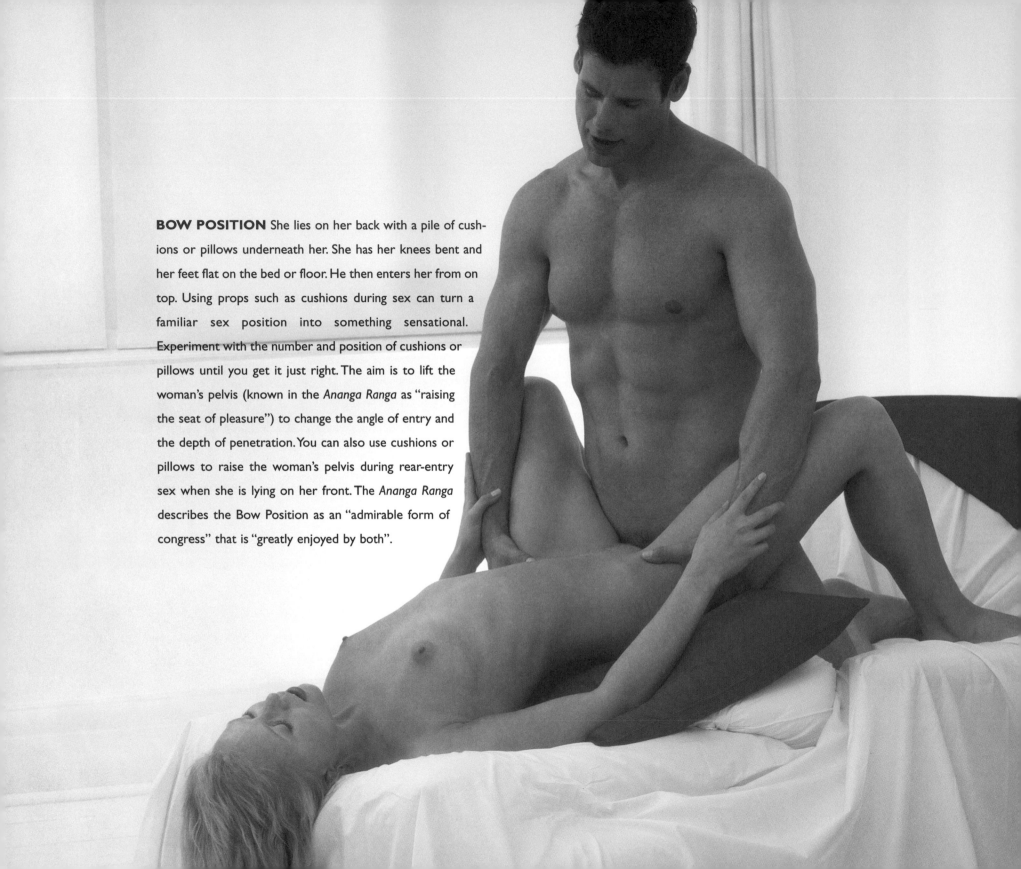

BOW POSITION She lies on her back with a pile of cushions or pillows underneath her. She has her knees bent and her feet flat on the bed or floor. He then enters her from on top. Using props such as cushions during sex can turn a familiar sex position into something sensational. Experiment with the number and position of cushions or pillows until you get it just right. The aim is to lift the woman's pelvis (known in the *Ananga Ranga* as "raising the seat of pleasure") to change the angle of entry and the depth of penetration. You can also use cushions or pillows to raise the woman's pelvis during rear-entry sex when she is lying on her front. The *Ananga Ranga* describes the Bow Position as an "admirable form of congress" that is "greatly enjoyed by both".

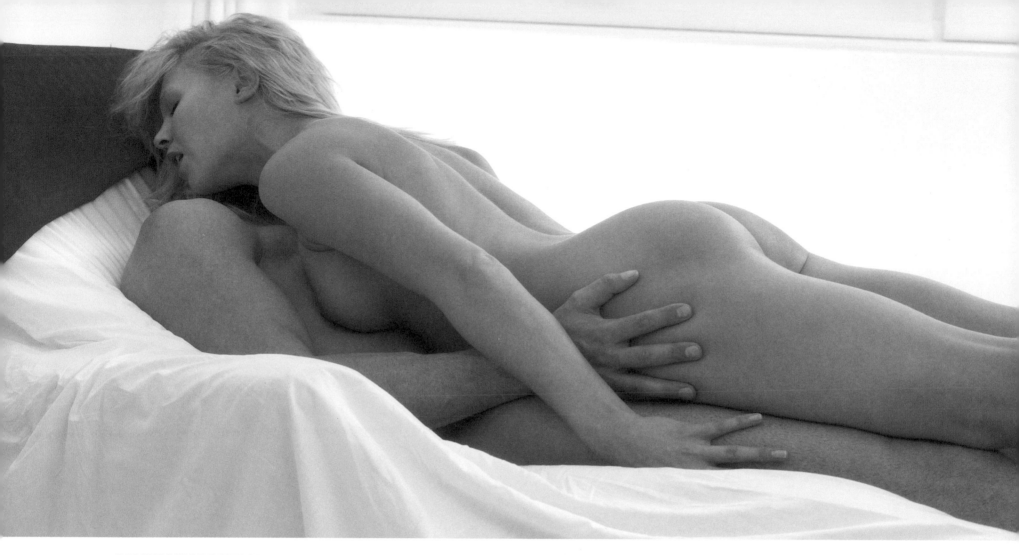

CONTRARY POSITION He lies on his back and she lies on top of him with her breasts against his chest and her hands on his waist. The *Ananga Ranga* then instructs the woman to enjoy her man by moving her hips sharply in a variety of directions. Meanwhile, the man can either lie still or guide the movement of her hips with his hands.

To support her weight better in this position, the woman can rest her hands either side of the man's body and put her feet on the tops of his feet, so that she can push against them. The higher up she lies on the man's body the more clitoral friction she receives when she moves against his pubic bone.

FAST AND PASSIONATE

These two standing positions from the *Ananga Ranga* are

perfect for sex that is driven by speed, urgency and passion.

The only drawback of standing positions is that women may

not receive the prolonged and rhythmic stimulation that they

need to reach orgasm. A good way of overcoming this is to

kneel down and give her oral sex before penetration or to

caress her clitoris straight afterwards. If there is space, and

you have the strength and the balance, you can move from

the Knee and Elbow Standing Form into a kneeling position

and then into a man-on-top position.

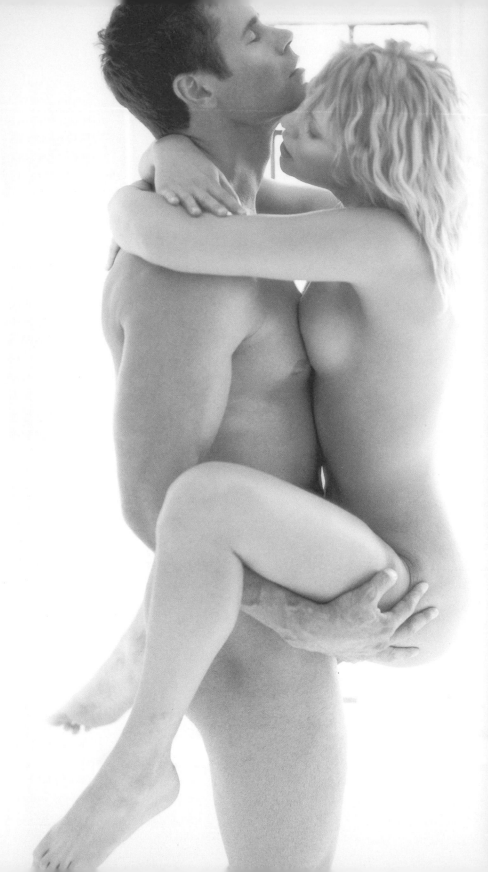

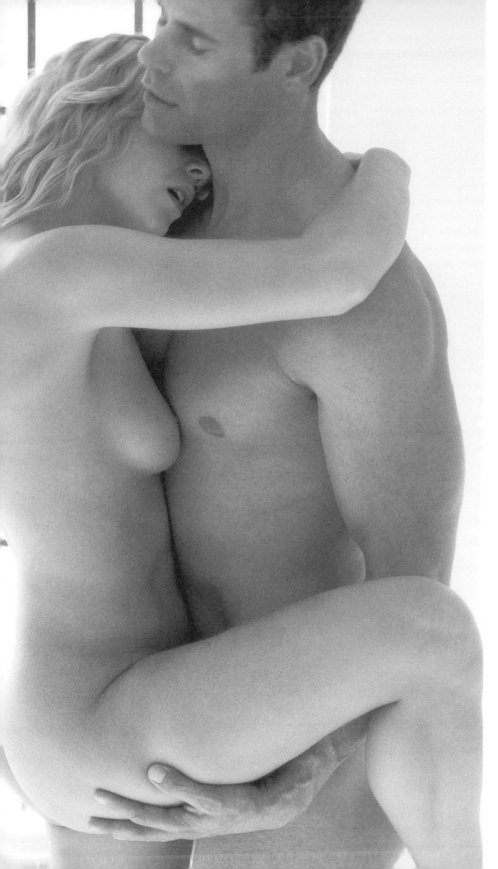

KNEE AND ELBOW STANDING FORM (far left) The man lifts the woman up so that her knees rest in the crooks of his elbows. She wraps her arms around his neck. Although this sex position demands a fair amount of endurance from the man, it has a very secure quality once you're in it. The feeling of being so completely held can be a huge turn-on for women, and men can enjoy the assertive display of masculine strength. Even if you can't hold this pose for a long time, it's fun to try between other sex positions and it's a sexy way of travelling – for example, if you're moving from the living room to the bedroom.

LEG RAISE (left) There's something effortlessly casual about this position in which she presses her body to his and raises one of her legs alongside his body for him to enter her. Depending on your respective heights (for example, if he's tall and she's petite), you may only be able to achieve fairly shallow penetration in this position. You can go deeper if he bends his knees into a semi-squat or if she stands on a slightly raised surface.

DEEP AND EROTIC

Of the following four sex positions from the *Ananga Ranga*, the Pressed-thigh Position offers the deepest penetration because the woman's legs are drawn up so closely to her body. The Elephant Pose combines the pleasure of feeling the penis high in the vagina with the raunchy animalism of rear-entry sex. The Large Bee is a woman-on-top position which means that she is in charge of the depth of penetration and the pace of lovemaking. Couples who relish the feeling of being deeply joined in a static position (great for Tantric sex) will enjoy the Cross-legged Position.

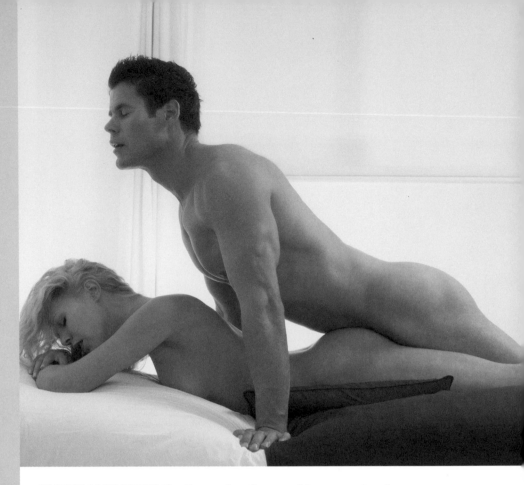

ELEPHANT POSE She lies on her front and he enters her from behind. You can increase the depth of penetration in this position in two ways. First, the woman can spread her legs very widely, and second, you can place one or more pillows or cushions under the woman's pelvis to make her vaginal entrance more accessible. Women can also enhance their enjoyment of this position by concentrating on the sensations emanating from the G-spot as the man massages the front wall of her vagina with his penis.

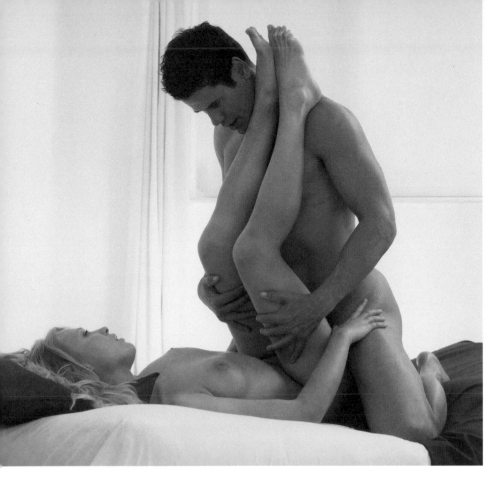

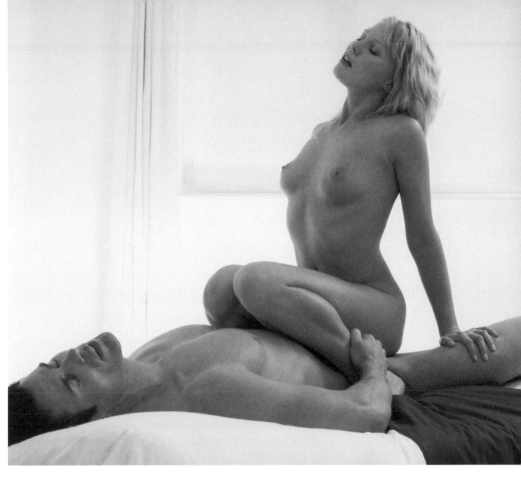

PRESSED-THIGH POSITION She lies on her back, raises her legs in the air and presses her thighs closely together. She can rest her legs over one of his shoulders or along the centre of his body. He can hold on to her thighs as he thrusts in and out of her or he can slide his hands underneath her buttocks and lift her up and down. Some women find it easier to contract their love muscles (see pages 22–3) tightly around the penis when their thighs are pressed together in this position – try it.

LARGE BEE He lies on his back and she lowers herself onto him in a squatting position (she is described as being like a large bee). Once he is inside her she closes her legs. The *Ananga Ranga* recommends that the woman satisfies herself in this position by "churning" – moving her waist in a circular motion. A variation of this position involves the woman opening her legs and leaning forward to place her hands on her lover's chest. Now she raises and lowers herself on his penis – he can use his hands to help guide her movements.

CROSS-LEGGED POSITION

Begin in a woman-on-top position: he lies on his back and she sits astride him. When you're ready to change position, he crosses his legs while lying down and pushes himself up into a sitting position. He keeps his legs crossed and she sits on his lap with her legs resting either side of him. He can place his hands on her shoulders. You can't move freely in this position, but it's wonderful for letting your bodies melt into each other and kissing passionately. If you enjoy using sex toys it's easy to incorporate a vibrator into this position; she can hold the tip against her clitoris. Alternatively, she can lie back on the bed and he can stimulate her with a vibrator or his hand.

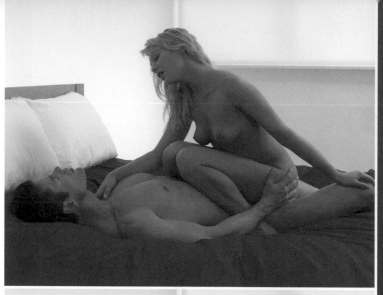

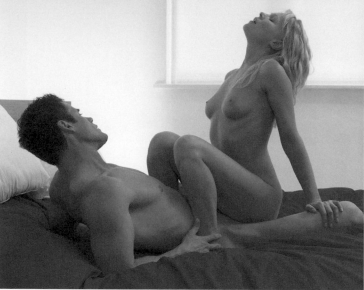

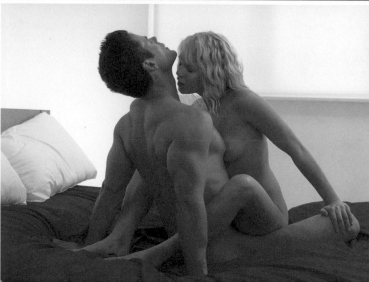

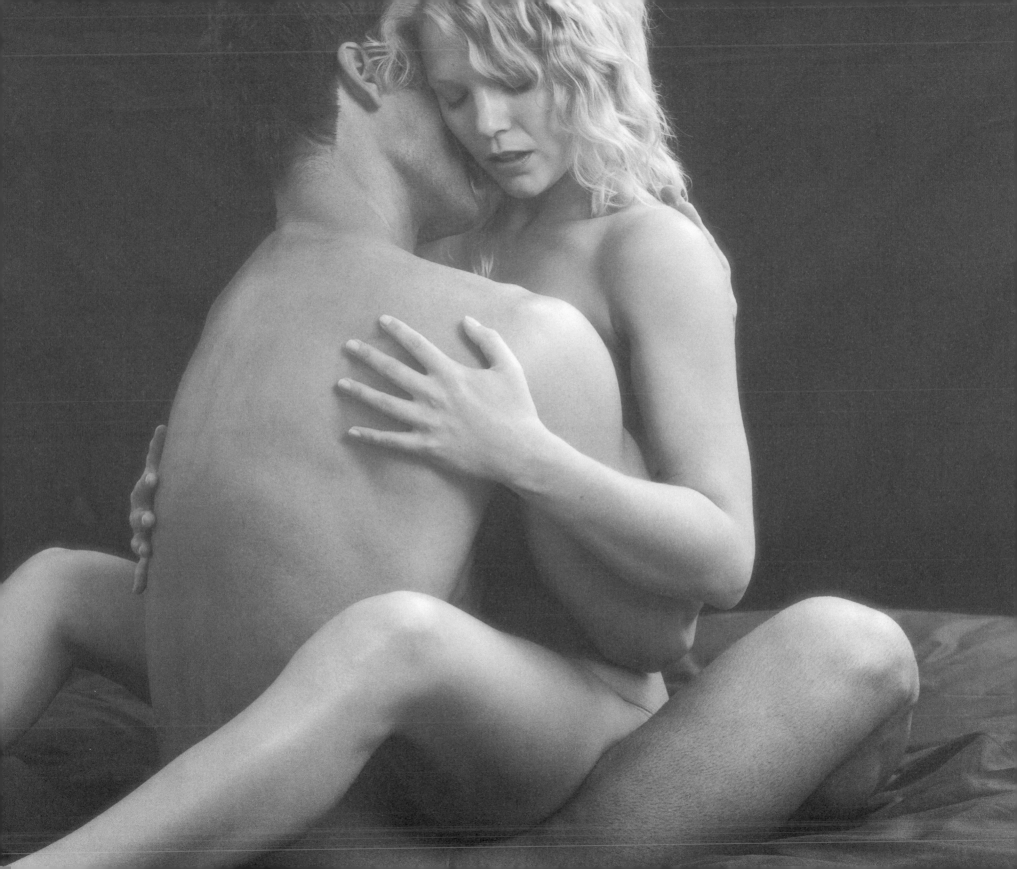

ADVENTUROUS

These two *Ananga Ranga* positions are best suited for small or light women or men with well-developed upper body strength. As its name suggests, the Lifting Position demands that the man lifts most of the woman's body weight during sex. In the Sitting-on-top Position, the woman's weight is concentrated around her lover's pelvis, although she can spread her weight by leaning back on her hands. Both these ways of making love present an interesting change from conventional man-on-top or woman-on-top positions – even if you can't keep going for very long, they're fun to try!

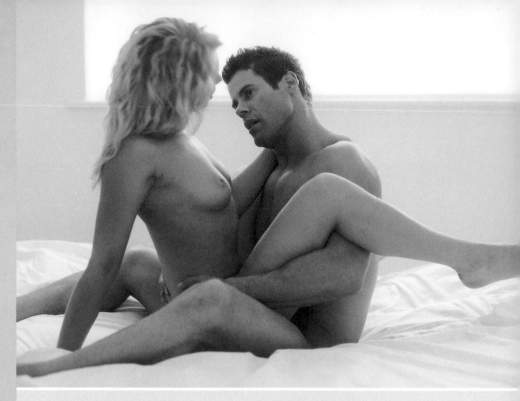

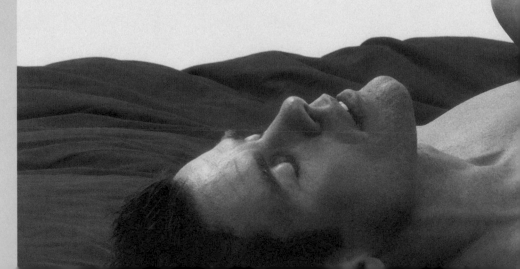

LIFTING POSITION (inset) He sits with his legs out in front of him and she sits on his lap with her legs hooked over his elbows. Her feet are off the floor or bed and he holds her body with his hands. The *Ananga Ranga* suggests that the man lifts the woman and moves her from left to right on his penis (but not up or down) until the "supreme moment". The woman can support some of her body weight by leaning back on her hands.

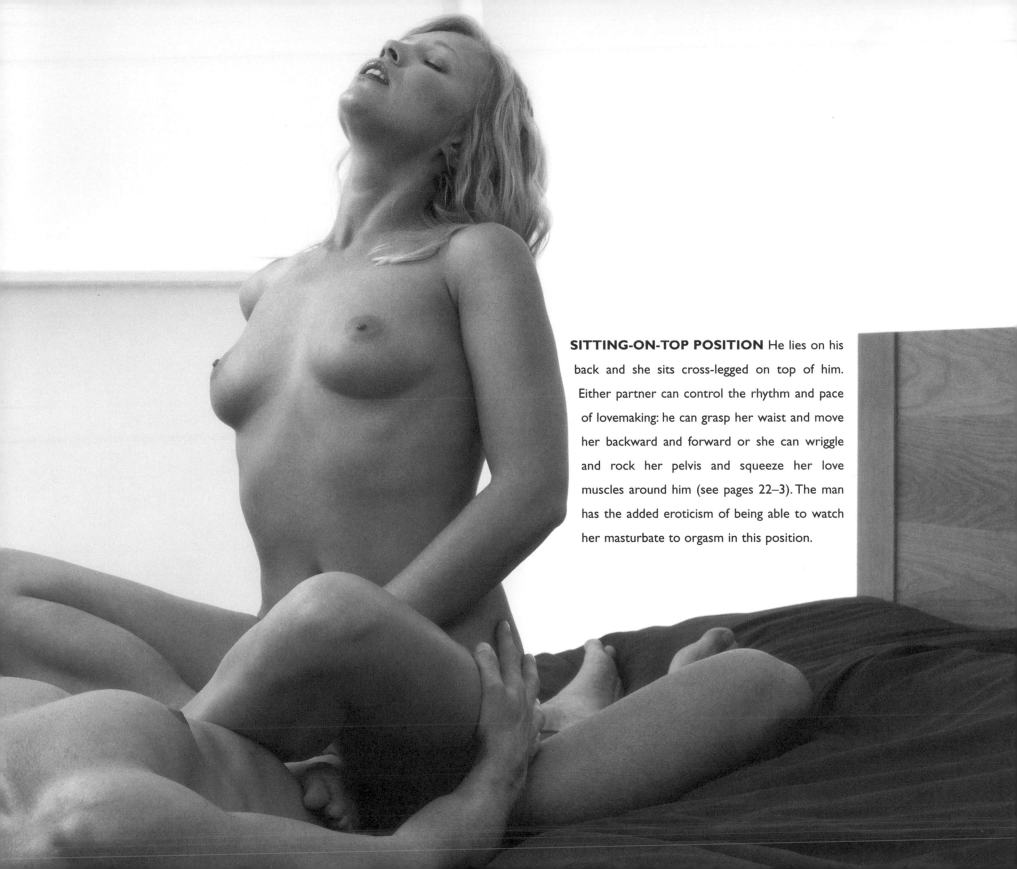

SITTING-ON-TOP POSITION He lies on his back and she sits cross-legged on top of him. Either partner can control the rhythm and pace of lovemaking: he can grasp her waist and move her backward and forward or she can wriggle and rock her pelvis and squeeze her love muscles around him (see pages 22–3). The man has the added eroticism of being able to watch her masturbate to orgasm in this position.

ANANGA RANGA SEQUENCE

This is a fairly restful sequence of sex positions, which you and your lover can flow into

one after the other without the need for him to withdraw. The first three positions are all

sitting up positions in which neither partner dominates. Then, in the next three positions,

the woman can take control by straddling, sitting or lying on top of the man – she can

control the pace of lovemaking and move in whatever way she wants. To do the final

three positions you roll over onto your sides into the Transverse Position and then the

Thigh Clasp. The climax of the sequence is the Pressed-thigh Position in which the

woman hooks her feet over his shoulders as he thrusts inside her.

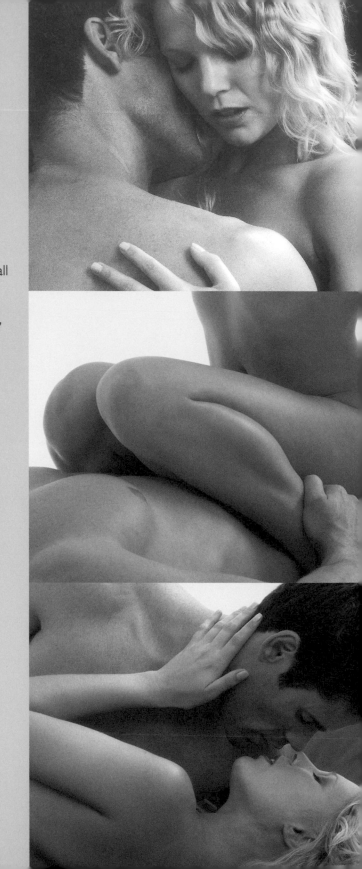

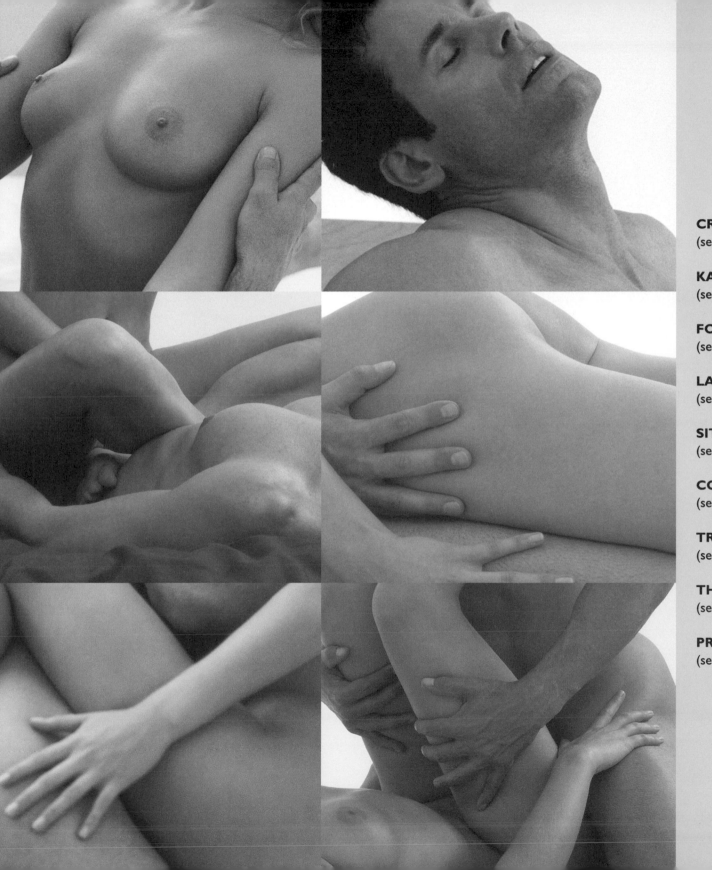

THE PERFUMED GARDEN POSITIONS

The author of *The Perfumed Garden*, Sheikh Nefzawi, gives instructions for 11 different sex positions entitled: First Posture, Second Posture, and so on. These are shown on the following pages. In addition there are 28 positions that Nefzawi borrows from the Hindus. Some of these are omitted here as they are impossible to perform without specially designed equipment – for example, the Hanging Posture demands that the woman is suspended by cords from the ceiling and raised and lowered by a pulley; or because they are very similar to another position – for example, the Sheep's Posture differs from the Sixth Posture only in that the woman rests on her forearms rather than her elbows.

Nefzawi describes sexual union as man's highest pleasure. Connoisseurs of copulation should experiment with as many different postures as possible in order to learn which ones give the greatest pleasure. And as Nefzawi says, if anyone thinks that the number of sex positions presented in his text is too small, then it is up to lovers to invent more! But just as important as mastering different positions is the attention that lovers give to embracing, kissing and sucking one another's lips – Nefzawi believes this is a true source of happiness and satisfaction for both the man and the woman.

The way in which you end sex is also an important skill that we should practise: Nefzawi advocates that rather than withdrawing his member abruptly after ejaculation, the man should withdraw gently and rest with his lover while lying on his right side. If you're planning to have sex a second time, you should perfume yourself with sweet fragrances and then begin all over again!

SLOW AND SOULFUL

These six positions from *The Perfumed Garden* are all face-to-face postures that create strong feelings of bondedness and intimacy between you and your lover. Some of the positions are similar to the missionary position, such as the First Posture. Others are more unusual, such as The Jointer, in which you and your lover sit upright with your legs entwined and move backward and forward in time with each other. In all of the following positions you can be close enough for a full-body hug and far enough apart to move and thrust against each other.

FIRST POSTURE She lies on her back and raises her legs with her knees bent, he then penetrates her from on top. This classic position is a staple in many couples' sex lives. It's an easy and comfortable way of making love: he can move freely inside her, she can focus on the building intensity of genital sensations as he thrusts, and both of you can enjoy looking at each other's face. To introduce new sensations she can move her knees wider apart or raise or lower her legs.

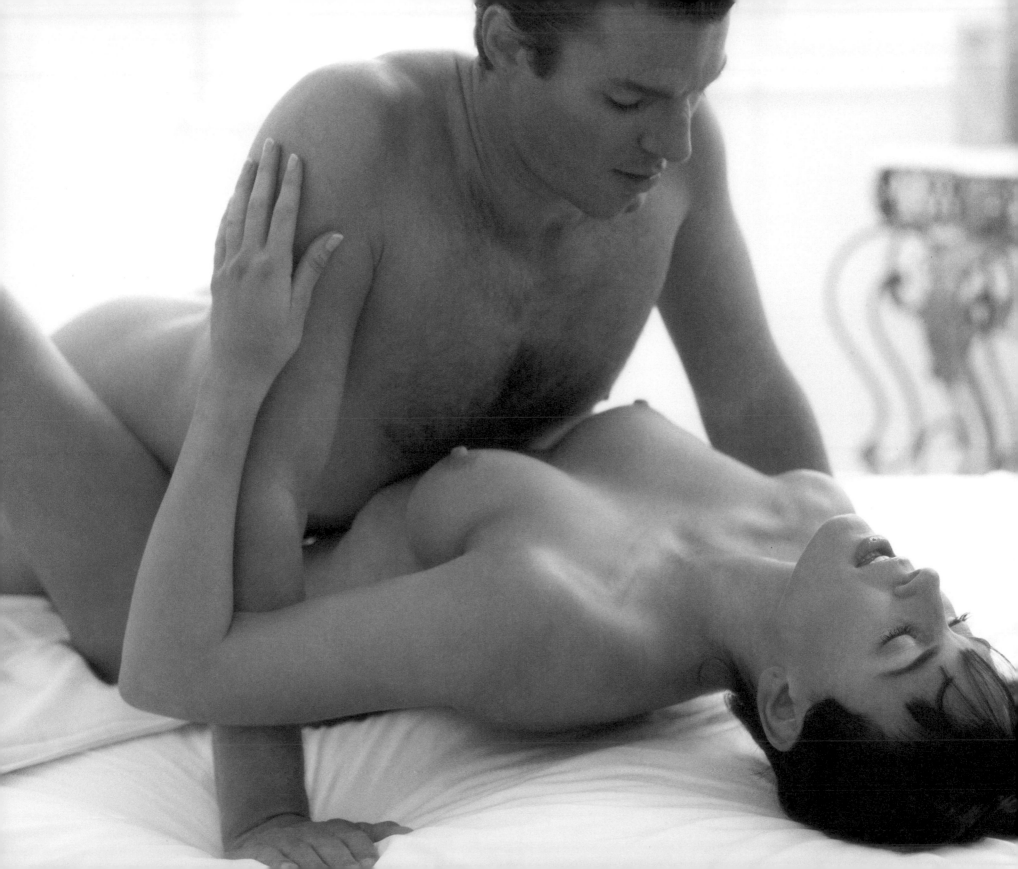

FIFTH POSTURE (right) She lies on her side and he positions himself between her thighs and enters her. Side-by-side sex positions like this are great for lazy lovemaking when neither of you feels like being on top. If you're having sex on the floor, the Fifth Posture can be the start of a dynamic sequence of positions: start in this posture and then roll into a man-on-top position, such as the First Posture, and then over again into a woman-on-top position. From here the woman can sit up and the man can stimulate her clitoris with his hand. The Fifth Posture is also a loving, peaceful position to lie and talk in after you have finished making love.

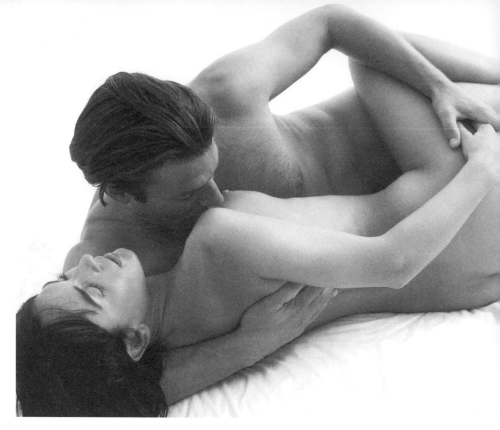

EIGHTH POSTURE (right) She lies on her back and he kneels astride her. Unlike many other man-on-top positions, the man cannot penetrate the woman freely in this posture because her legs are inside rather than outside his. What he can do is hold his erect penis in his hand and guide it in and out of her vaginal entrance and rub his glans in rhythmic circles around her clitoris. This is deeply arousing for both of you — when you're really turned on you can move into a position that allows greater freedom of movement.

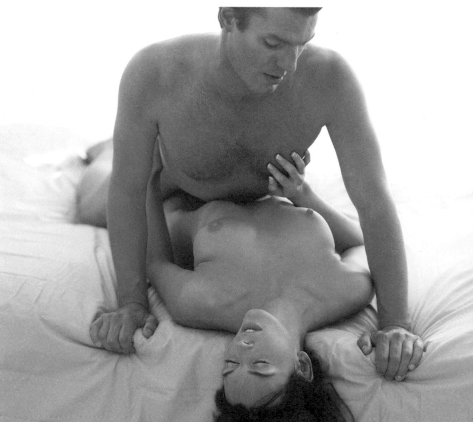

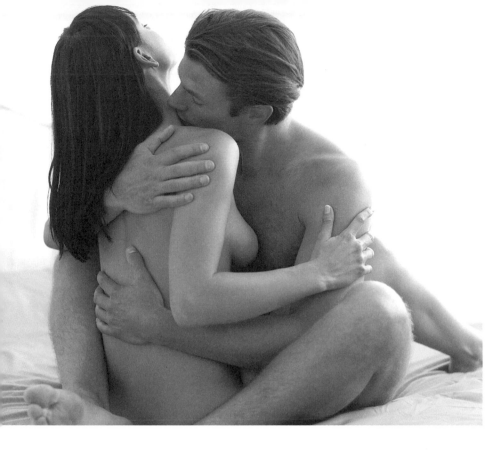

THE JOINTER (left) You both sit facing each other on a bed or the floor and the woman puts her right thigh over the man's left thigh. He then puts his right thigh over her left thigh and you grasp hold of each other. Nefzawi instructs couples to move in a see-saw motion taking turns to lean backward and forward in time with the movements of the penis in the vagina.

THE FUSION OF LOVE (left) She lies on her right side and he lies on his left side. She puts her top leg over his hip and he stretches his top leg between her legs. This is a gentle and intimate position that is great for slow lovemaking interspersed with plenty of tender kissing. You can get into this position after she has given him oral sex – she simply slides up his body. To up the erotic tempo during side-by-side sex, try scratching each other's buttocks with your fingernails or sucking each other's fingers in the same rhythm that his penis enters her vagina.

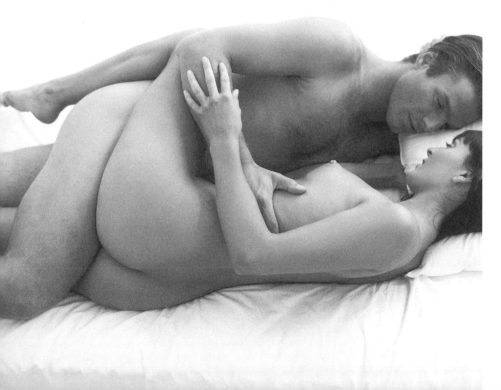

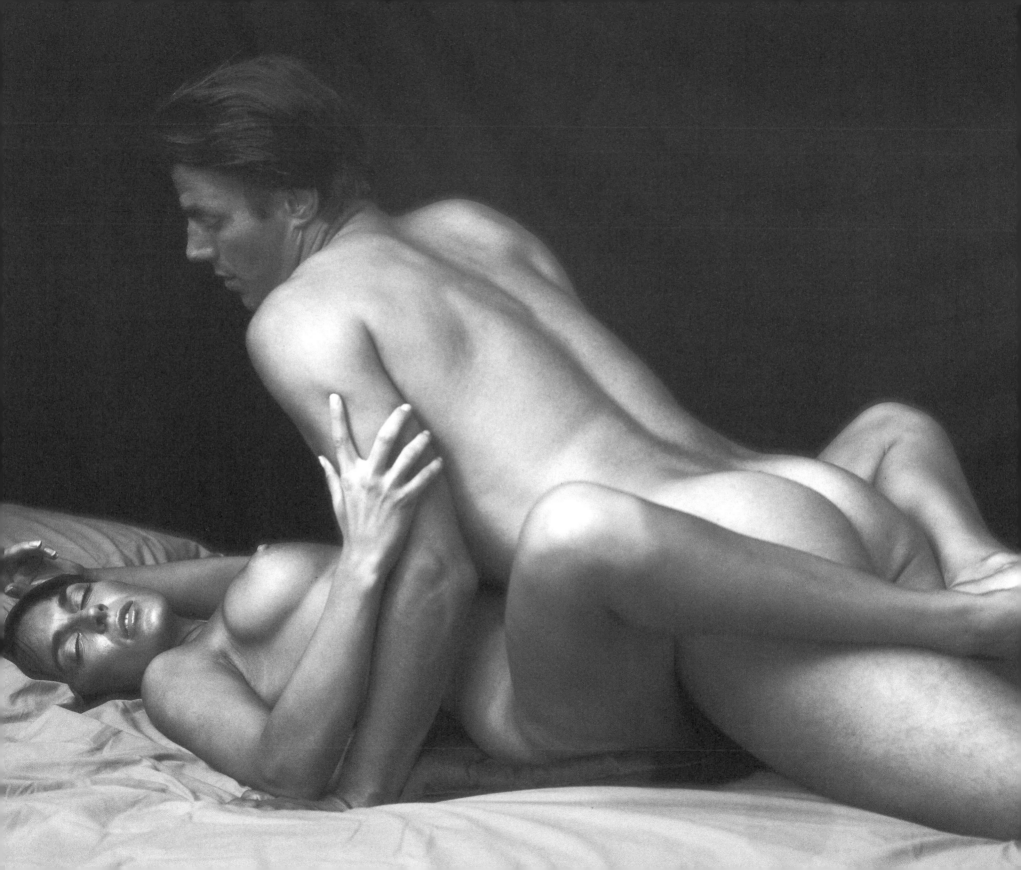

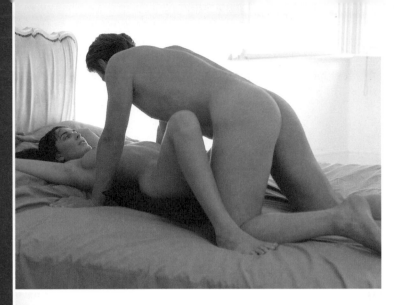

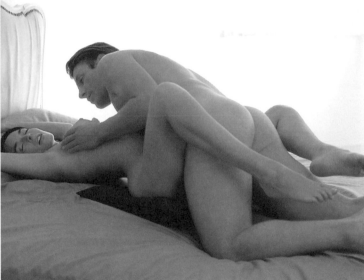

ELEVENTH POSTURE She lies on her back with one or more cushions or pillows under her buttocks, then she lets her knees fall to the sides and presses the soles of her feet together. Now the man gets on top and enters her. A variation of this posture is for the woman to press the soles of her feet together after the man has penetrated her – this may be more comfortable as her feet rest on the backs of his legs. If the man presses his pelvis tightly against the woman during sex, her clitoris receives lots of friction as he thrusts.

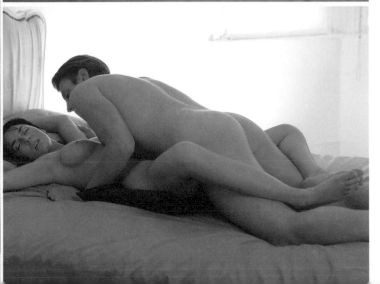

FAST AND PASSIONATE

Try these three sex positions from *The Perfumed Garden* for

times when you want sex that is immediate, impulsive and

unplanned. For sex at a second's notice, go for Belly to Belly

in which the man enters his lover simply by standing in front

of her. Or try Driving in the Peg for sex in which the woman

is literally swept off her feet. The Ninth Posture captures the

exciting, animalistic feeling of the Doggy Pose, but it is more

restful because you are supported by cushions or pillows.

Make up variations of these positions to create your own

personal repertoire for fast and passionate sex.

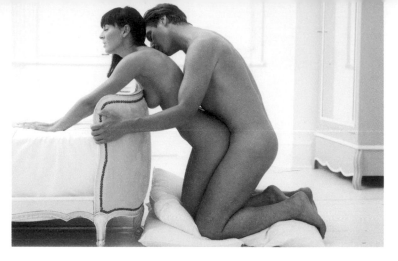

NINTH POSTURE (above) Both partners kneel on the floor on a pile of cushions or pillows. She leans forward over a bed or sofa as he enters her from behind. He can alternate between shallow and deep thrusts. Be uninhibited and make as much noise as you want to!

BELLY TO BELLY (right) You stand face-to-face with your hands around each other's waist. She has her feet wide apart and he has his feet between hers. If couples are a similar height, this can be one of the most erotic positions because you can get into it so quickly. If she is much shorter than him, she can try standing on a raised surface.

DRIVING IN THE PEG (far right) He lifts her up and she puts her arms around his neck and her legs around his waist. She puts her feet on a wall behind her to support some of her weight. He puts his hands around her waist and guides her body. If this position gets tiring, the man can turn around so that the woman's back rests against the wall – a great position for a passionate mid-sex kiss.

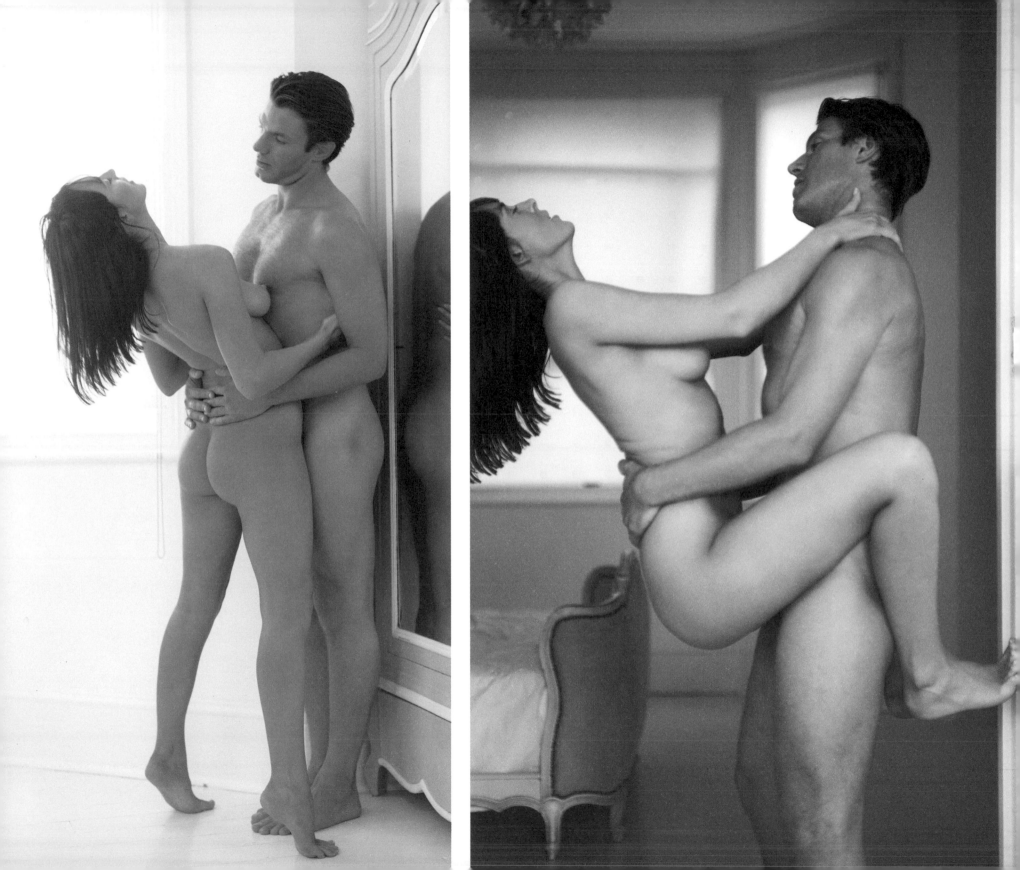

DEEP AND EROTIC

This selection from *The Perfumed Garden* comprises two face-to-face and two rear-entry positions. The Second Posture offers the deepest penetration while the Fourth Posture combines deep penetration with intimacy and lots of skin-to-skin contact. The Mutual View of the Buttocks combines deep penetration with female dominance plus the deeply erotic pleasure of watching the penis entering the vagina. A more familiar position, which lots of couples love for passion and maximum penetration, is the Sixth Posture, also known as the Doggy Pose.

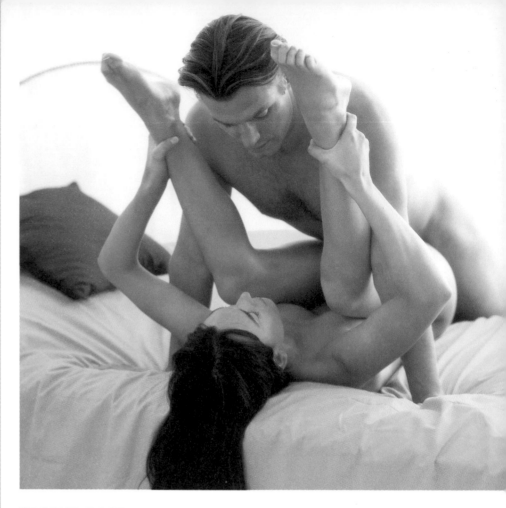

SECOND POSTURE This position demands a lot of suppleness from the woman: she lies on her back and raises her legs so that her toes are over her ears (or as close to her ears as she can get them). He gets on top and enters her. Nefzawi recommends this position for men with a short member. Well-endowed men should move very gently in the Second Posture because the vagina is contracted and vigorous thrusting can be uncomfortable.

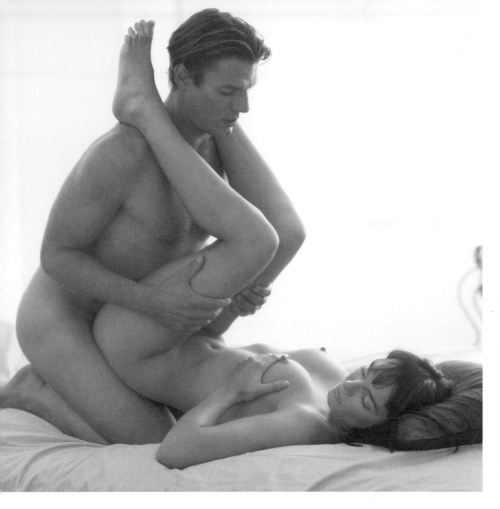

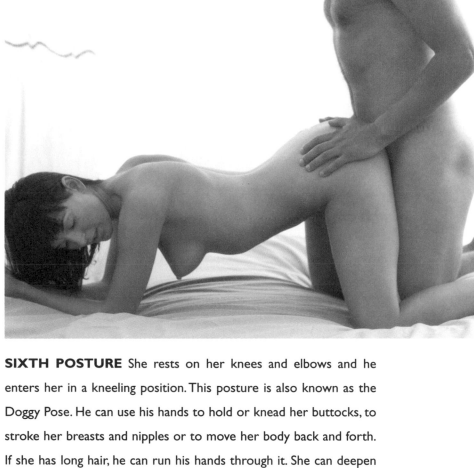

FOURTH POSTURE She lies on her back and puts her legs over his shoulders. Her lower body rests along the front of his thighs so that her pelvis is raised. As Nefzawi says, the man's penis is exactly opposite the woman's vulva in this position. He can hold onto her legs and she can use her hands to caress his thighs, stroke her breasts or stimulate her clitoris. As he moves inside her he can ask for guidance about which speed and depth best stimulates her G-spot.

SIXTH POSTURE She rests on her knees and elbows and he enters her in a kneeling position. This posture is also known as the Doggy Pose. He can use his hands to hold or knead her buttocks, to stroke her breasts and nipples or to move her body back and forth. If she has long hair, he can run his hands through it. She can deepen penetration by lowering her upper body to the floor or make it more shallow by kneeling upright so that her body is parallel to his.

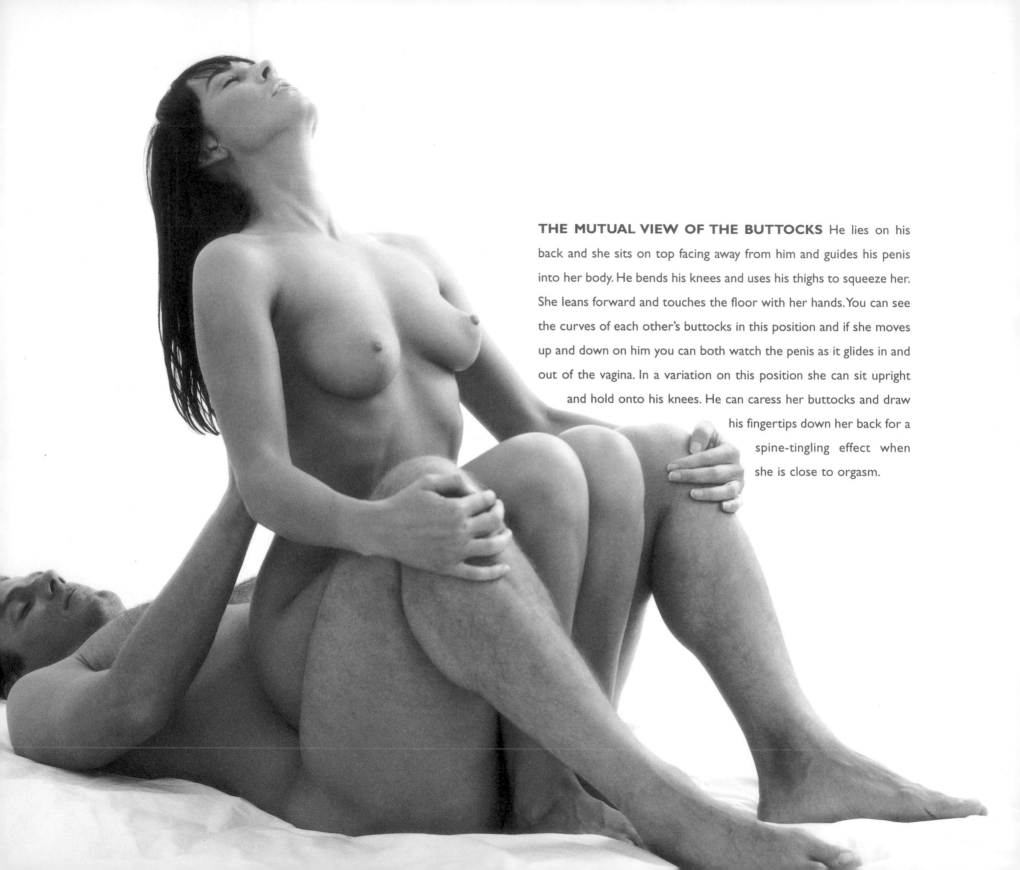

THE MUTUAL VIEW OF THE BUTTOCKS He lies on his back and she sits on top facing away from him and guides his penis into her body. He bends his knees and uses his thighs to squeeze her. She leans forward and touches the floor with her hands. You can see the curves of each other's buttocks in this position and if she moves up and down on him you can both watch the penis as it glides in and out of the vagina. In a variation on this position she can sit upright and hold onto his knees. He can caress her buttocks and draw his fingertips down her back for a spine-tingling effect when she is close to orgasm.

ADVENTUROUS

These five positions from *The Perfumed Garden* are for love-making with novelty value for times when you and your partner are feeling especially creative. Some of the positions demand a lot of thigh strength, such as Riding the Member in which the woman squats over the man and raises and lowers herself on his penis. Other postures demand a degree of suppleness, such as the Seventh Posture in which the woman's legs are at right angles to each other. The most unusual of the positions is Drawing the Bow, a side-by-side position that defies categorization.

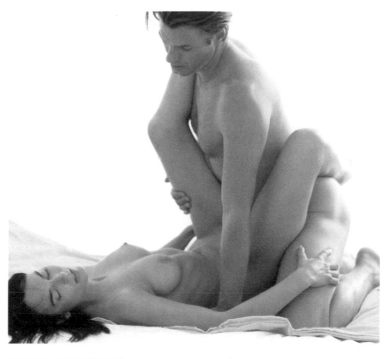

THIRD POSTURE He lies on top of her with one of her legs under his arm and her other leg over his shoulder. Although she doesn't have much freedom of movement she can wriggle her hips and contract her love muscles around his penis (see pages 22–3). It's also easy for her to touch her nipples and clitoris with her fingers in this position. Try experimenting with subtle changes of angle – for example, by putting cushions or pillows under her lower back or bringing the knee of her uppermost leg closer to her chest.

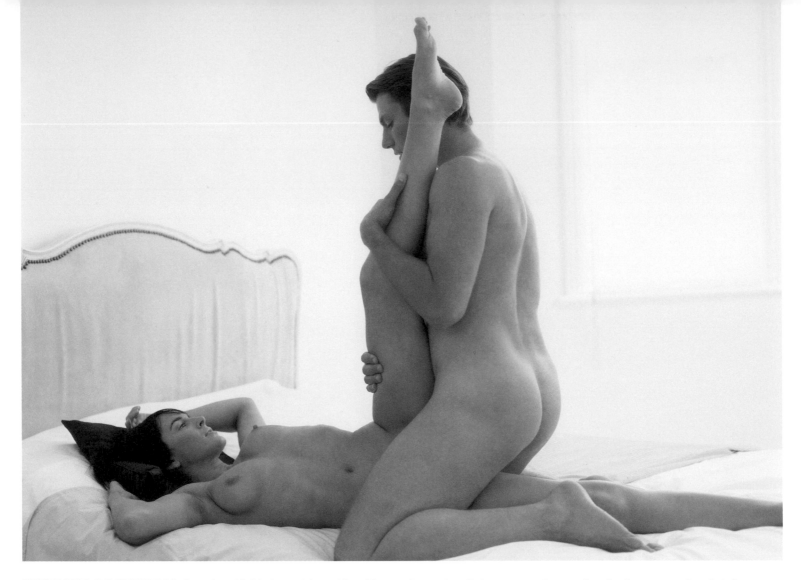

SEVENTH POSTURE He kneels with his legs either side of her outstretched leg. She then raises her free leg and rests it on his shoulder. Nefzawi specifies that penetration should take place with the woman on her side, but unless she is exceptionally supple it may be easier if the woman lies on her back or just tilts slightly to one side. If she wants to try the position on her side it can help if she grabs the foot of her raised leg and pulls it toward her body to make her vaginal entrance more accessible.

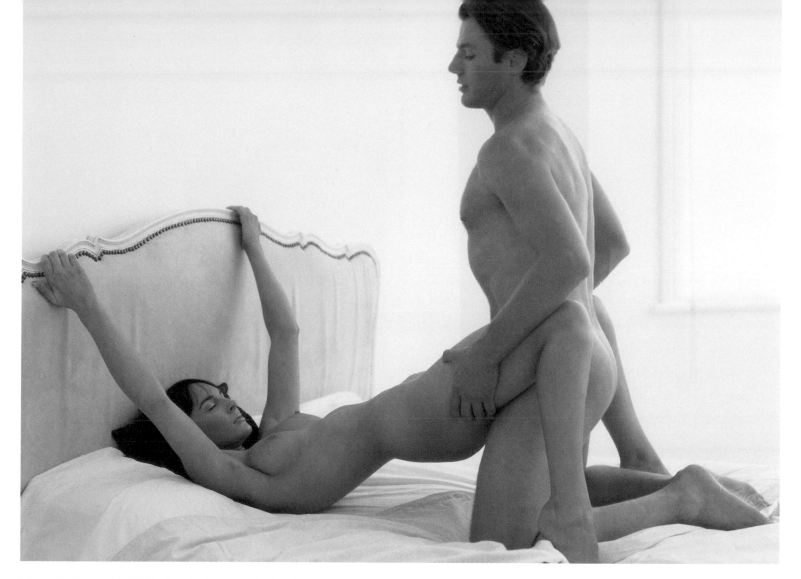

TENTH POSTURE She lies back on the bed and grasps the headboard firmly. Then she clasps his hips with her legs and he enters her, lifting up her pelvis as he does so. She uses her leg muscles to push and pull herself back and forth on his penis. He synchronizes his movements to the rhythm of hers. If it's difficult to move in this position, the woman can drop her hips back down onto the bed and the man can thrust more freely. If both of you hold the headboard, she feels the full force of his movements throughout her body.

RIDING THE MEMBER He lies down with a cushion under his shoulders and raises his knees toward his shoulders. She stands astride him and lowers herself onto his erect penis. Nefzawi describes two ways of moving in this position: either she moves up and down on him by bending her knees, or he moves her with his legs while she grasps his knees or shoulders for support. Women can enjoy being dominant in this position while men get to experience the eroticism of being ridden. In a variation you can try leaning in toward each other so that your faces are nearly touching – if both of you are supple, you will be able to kiss.

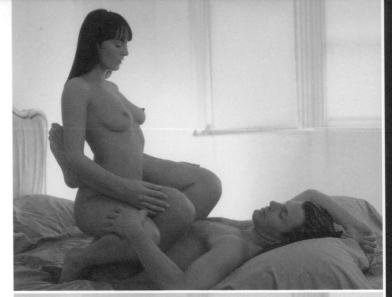
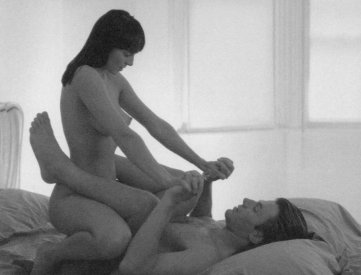
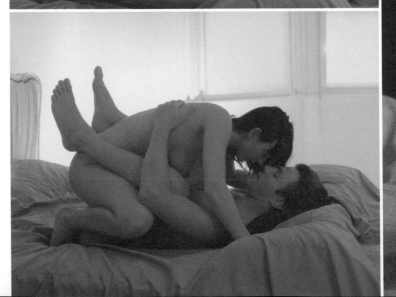

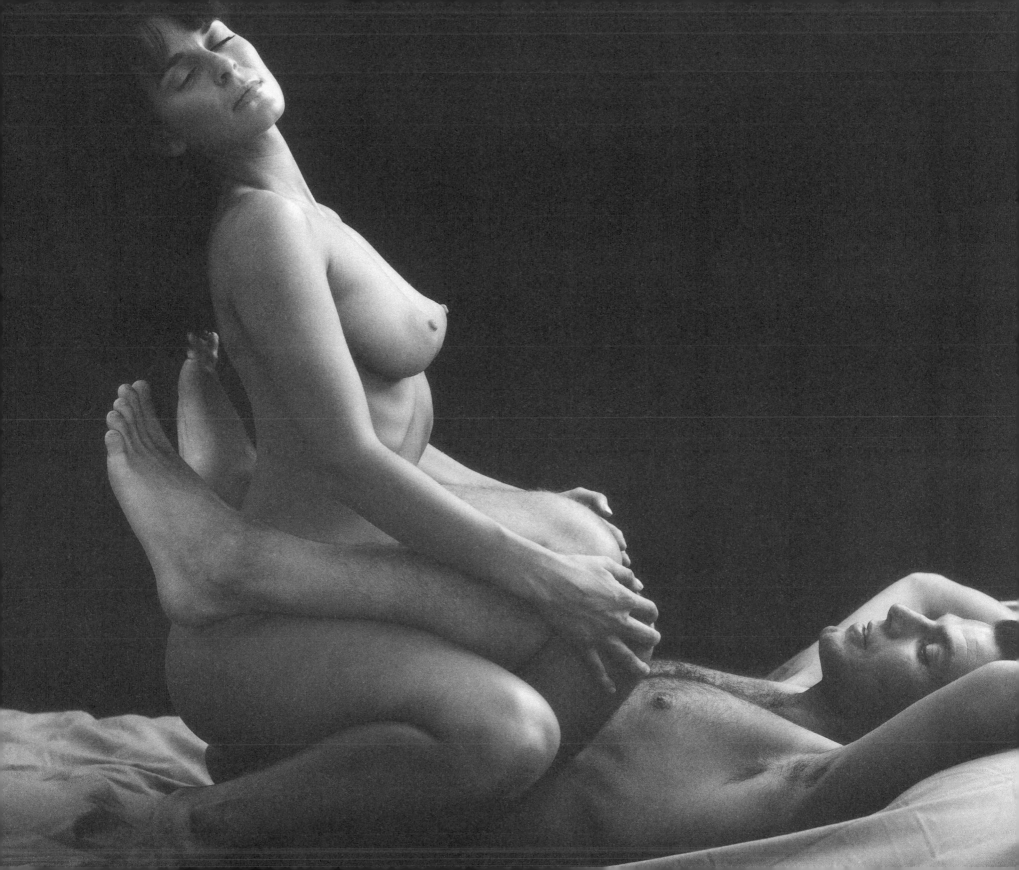

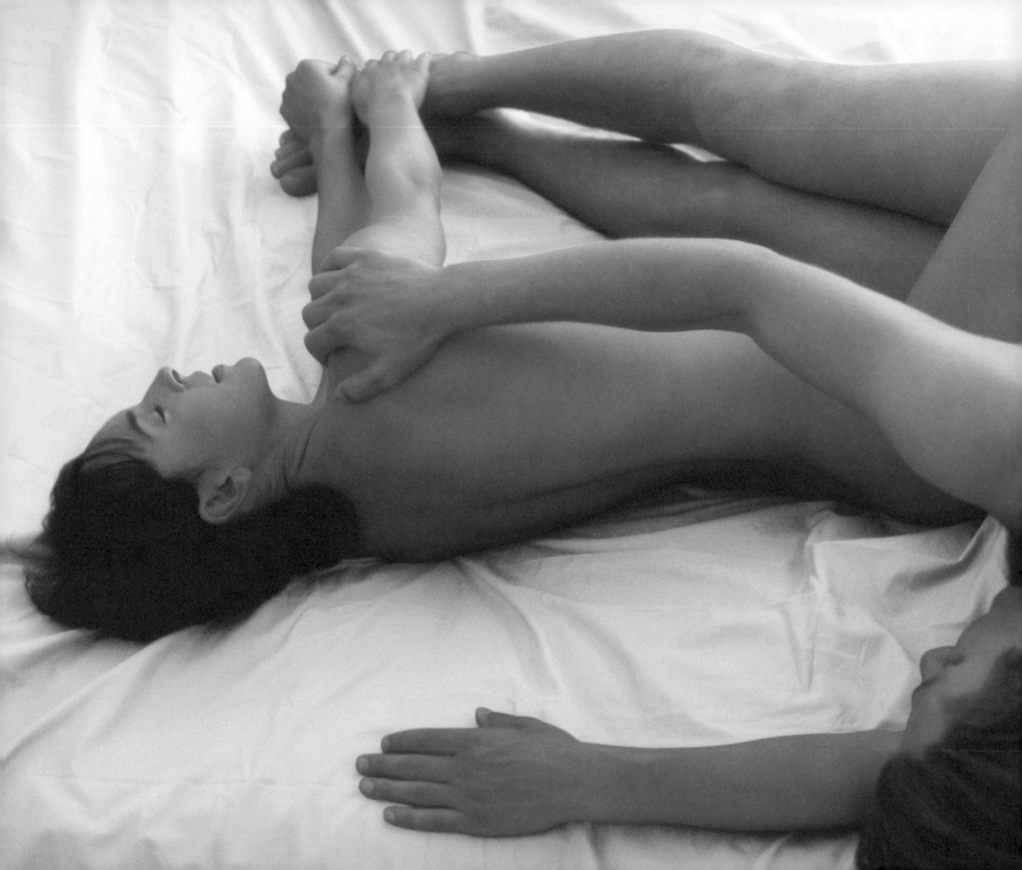

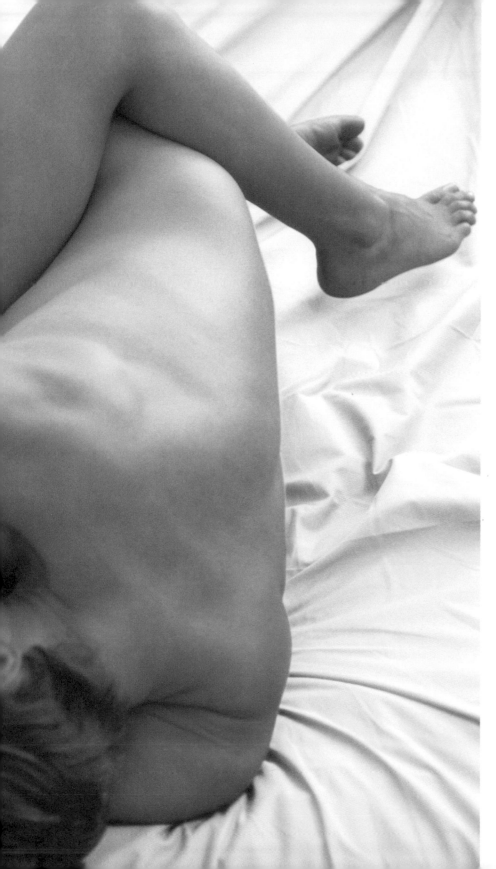

DRAWING THE BOW She lies on her side and he lies behind her between her legs. He puts one or both of his hands on her shoulders and she grasps his feet and pulls them toward her. Joined in this way you form the shape of a bow and arrow. The excitement of this position comes from its novelty. She can heighten sensation by squeezing and massaging his toes or he can run his fingers down the length of her back. If you feel a sense of freedom and anonymity in this position, make the most of it by indulging in a favourite fantasy.

THE PERFUMED GARDEN SEQUENCE

This sequence of sex positions begins with four rear-entry positions – with some expert

maneuvering you can do the first three one after the other without him withdrawing.

To move from the opening position into Drawing the Bow, she needs to lie down on

him, he then tightly embraces her and you both roll onto your sides. For the final

rear-entry position, you need to move from the bed to the floor. Then you need to

separate again so that he can penetrate her in a man-on-top position. The two final

standing positions are for fun – because they don't allow much freedom of movement,

you may want to come back down onto the floor afterwards.

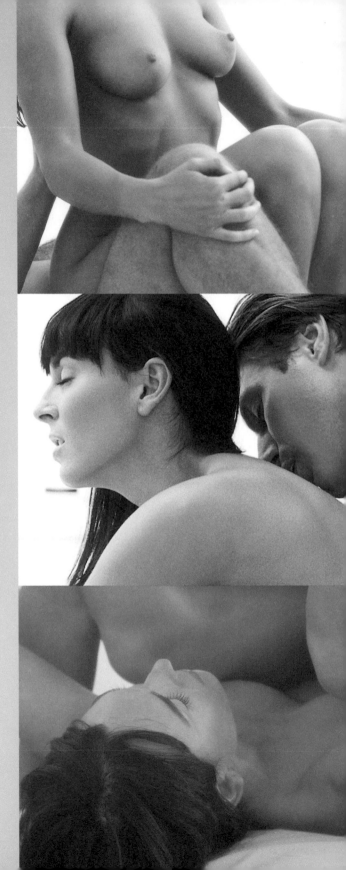

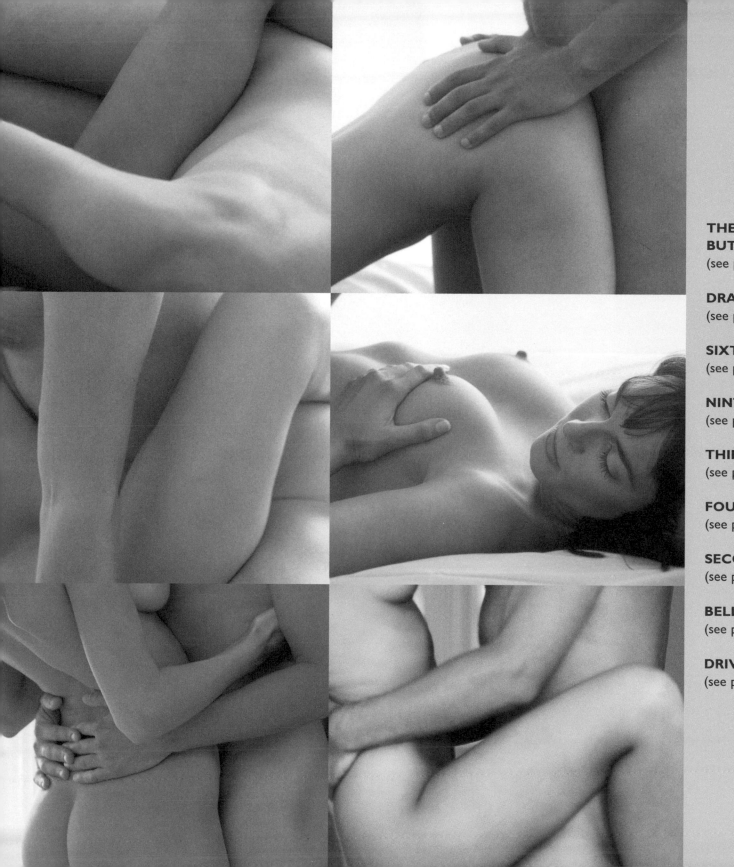

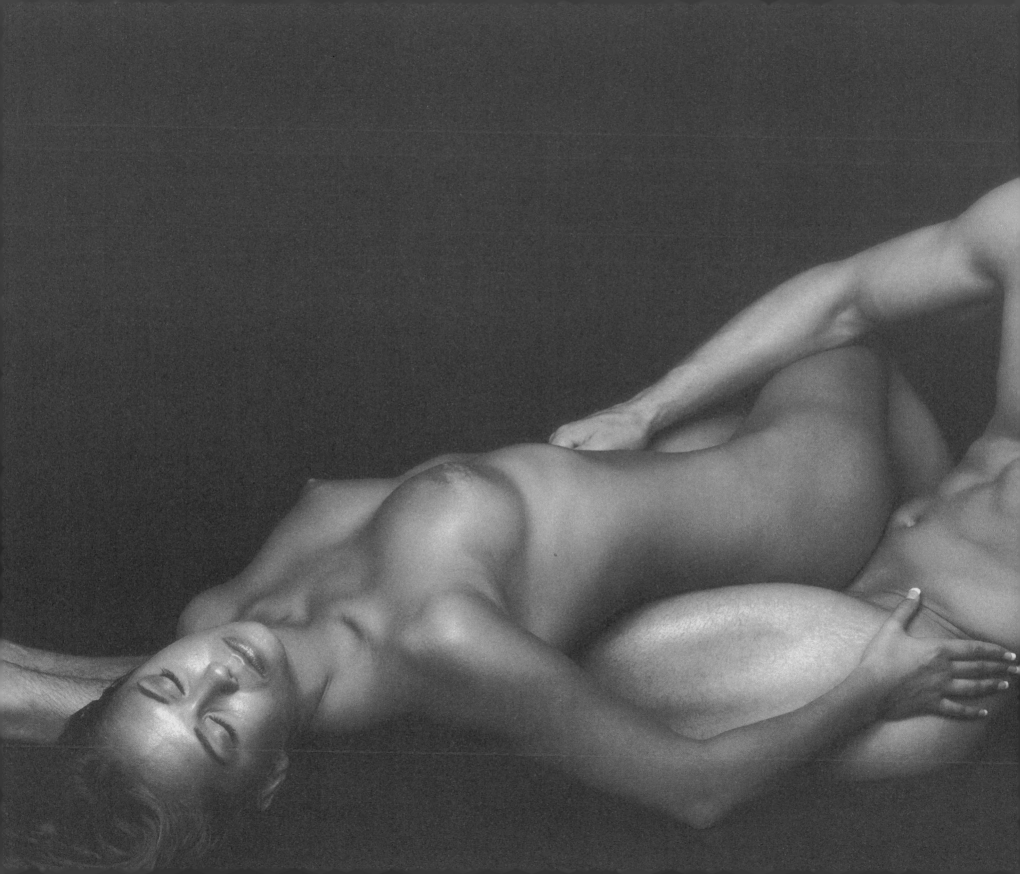

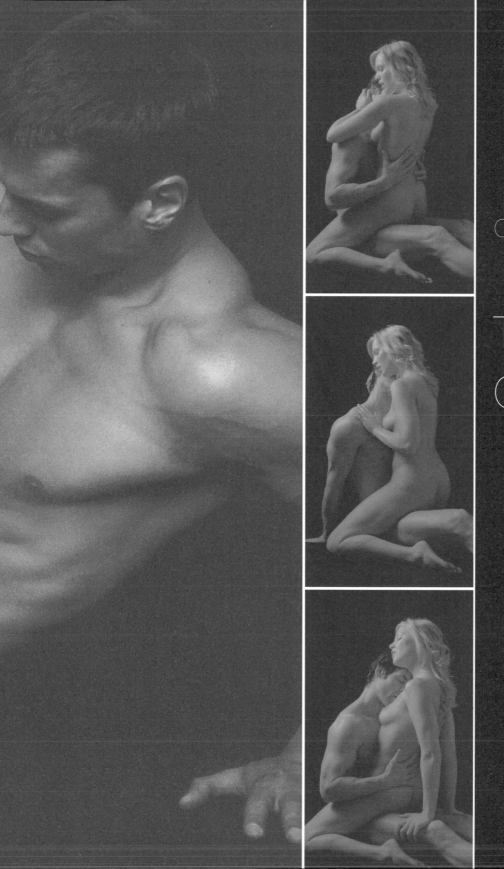

CHAPTER 4

THE TANTRA OF ECSTASY

THE TANTRIC PATH

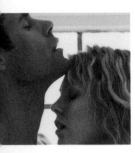

The ancient Indian art of Tantra is often perceived as a route to new levels of sexual ecstasy. Ultimately, this can be true for many Tantric practioners, but it's also true that Tantric practices take dedication, and rarely yield results overnight. Tantric sex involves overcoming a goal- and performance-oriented approach to sex and treating it as a route to spiritual transformation; a way of reaching a meditative and expanded state of mind.

Tantra philosophy centres around the erotic union of the Hindu god Shiva and goddess Shakti, which Hindus believe led to the creation of the universe. Men are seen as manifestations of Shiva and women as manifestations of Shakti. The combination of masculine and feminine energies that takes place during sexual intercourse is key to spiritual enlightenment.

UNLEARNING SEXUAL HABITS

Before embarking on a Tantric path it's necessary to overcome some myths about sex and unlearn some sexual habits. The Western approach to sex emphasizes that sex is successful only when the man has a strong, sustained erection and both lovers find it easy to reach a powerful genital orgasm as a result of intercourse. In Tantric sex arousal levels (and erections) are allowed to go up and down; stillness and minimal movements are valued more than vigorous thrusting; and cultivating a blissful expansion of energy inside the body is considered to be more important than orgasm. Try to let go of the idea that you must perform to a certain level or have a beautiful, thin, young or toned body. The more you put aside your expectations of what sex is about, the more free you will be to explore the subtle sensations that arise spontaneously inside you.

HONOURING YOUR PARTNER

Tantric teachers often suggest that you begin a Tantric practice by honouring your partner as a way of respecting the divine in each other. This could mean bowing to one another with your hands pressed together in prayer position, or making a sexual vow (see page 123). Even if you feel strange or silly doing some of the Tantric practices in this chapter, persevere with them – if necessary allow yourself to laugh or giggle and then carry on.

LOOKING INTO THE SOUL

Making eye contact with your lover is important during many Tantric practices. Rather than simply staring at your lover, use your mutual gazing to get into a meditative state of mind. Relax and connect with your partner by sharing a bath and doing the Conscious Kissing exercise on page 139. Now sit opposite each other and close your eyes. Synchronize your breathing. When you both feel ready, open your eyes and look into each other's left eye (which is considered to be more receptive than the right eye). Let yourself relax into the gaze – smile if you want to and then let the smile fade.

Bond with your lover through your gaze. Think to yourself: "I am giving and receiving love through my eyes" or simply repeat "I love you" inside your head like a mantra. Don't speak during this exercise. If you feel uncomfortable or self-conscious, acknowledge your feelings and then try to let them float away. If you get distracted keep bringing your attention back to your synchronized breathing or to the loving energy that is flowing between you and your partner.

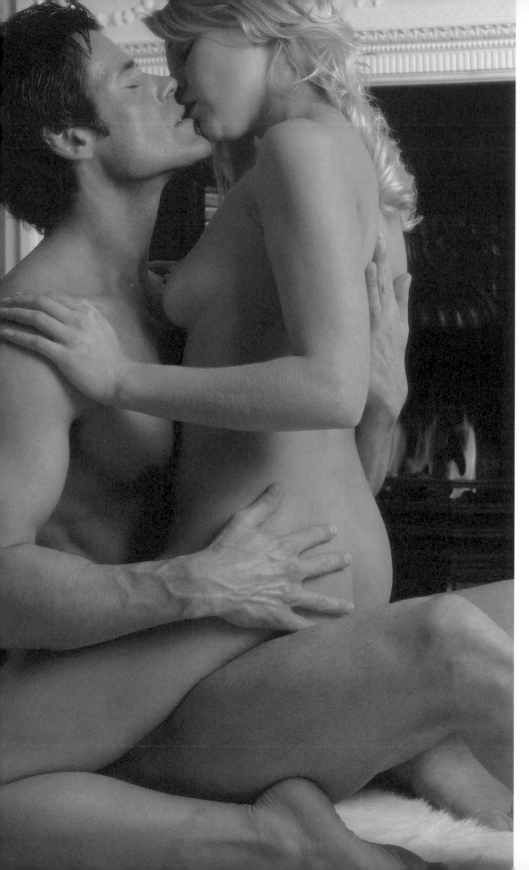

SEXUAL TRUST

The practices of Tantric sex require a lot of trust between you and your partner. You need to feel open and vulnerable with one another rather than fearful and defended. But to many people dropping their defences feels like an emotionally risky experience that they would rather avoid.

INTIMACY BY DEGREES

Emotional trust happens by degrees. If you make your partner feel loved and accepted, and if you feel loved and accepted in return, over time intimacy will blossom naturally in your relationship.

Hostility and criticism threaten intimacy. The first response most people have to criticism is to defend themselves or to criticize back. And if you're locked into the need to attack or defend, you will find it difficult to open yourself emotionally.

This is why it's crucial to suspend criticism in sexual relationships and specifically criticism about sex itself. If there's something you don't like about your sex life, rather than blaming your lover, recast what you want to say in a neutral or a positive way. For example, saying "I don't like the way you kiss me" will make your partner feel defensive and inadequate, whereas saying "I love it when we kiss each other gently on the lips before getting passionate" gives your partner clear guidance about what you enjoy. It also turns kissing into a joint responsibility.

FEAR OF FAILURE

If you and your lover feel that you must both put on a flawless sexual performance for one another, it becomes harder to be experimental because you are in fear of failure. You can develop sexual trust by accepting that not every sexual experience will go how you want it to, and supporting each other when this happens. If you can discuss sex impartially and even laugh about it, you will feel much more free to explore sex together.

Tell each other what you love most about sex. If you experienced something special during sex, don't keep it to yourself – describe in detail how you felt, what you were thinking at the time and what it meant to you. If you want to embark on a path of Tantric sex, sharing your deepest thoughts and feelings in this way is a route to a profound level of connection.

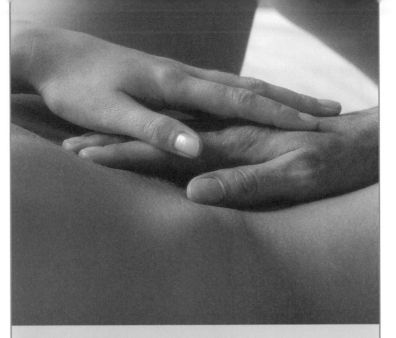

SEXUAL VOWS

Before you and your partner begin any Tantric sex practice, you can create an atmosphere of trust and intimacy by both speaking aloud an affirmation or vow that has personal relevance to you and your partner. Try making up a special vow together. Here are some examples:

• I love and honour you.

• Sex joins us emotionally and spiritually as well as physically.

• I will share my deepest thoughts and feelings with you.

• I want to share myself with you.

• I trust you.

• If sex goes wrong, we'll talk about it uncritically.

• I respect the sexual differences that exist between us.

• We are here together because we love each other.

SACRED SPACES

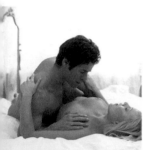

Tantric sex is about surrendering to the moment and letting your senses expand. Tantric teachers recommend creating a special sanctuary with your lover in which you feel safe and inspired.

CHOOSING A SPACE

According to the *Ananga Ranga*, the best room for sex is the largest, finest and most airy one. It should be purified with white-wash, decorated with pictures, and mirrors should be placed to reflect light. You may not be able to achieve the perfect space, but try to pick the largest room in your home – sex doesn't have to be confined to the bedroom – so that you can move freely, and dance (see page 37) if you want to.

BAN TECHNOLOGY

Technology is no longer confined to living rooms and studies – it's now common to find computers, telephones and televisions all over the home. Being surrounded by technology that buzzes, hums, bleeps or rings creates a kind of invisible stress upon us. It's important to remove every piece of technology that

connects you to the outside world from your chosen room. Remember – the level of surrender involved in Tantric sex is completely incompatible with a bleeping cell phone!

DECORATING A SPACE

Clutter also distracts the mind and creates a subtle but ever-present stress. Clear your space of things that you don't need or things that you no longer take pleasure in. Now clean the space.

Once you have created a blank canvas, consider what objects you would like to have around you: you might like to select beautiful paintings, sculptures, wall hangings or fabrics, or objects from nature, such as shells, flowers or stones. Choose things that have personal meaning for you and your lover.

If your sacred space is not in your bedroom, arrange some cushions and throws on the floor on which you can lie down. Light candles, scatter petals and burn incense (use the suggestions on page 12). Your aim is to transform a familiar room into a space that feels extraordinary or magical. When you enter the space, your spirits should lift.

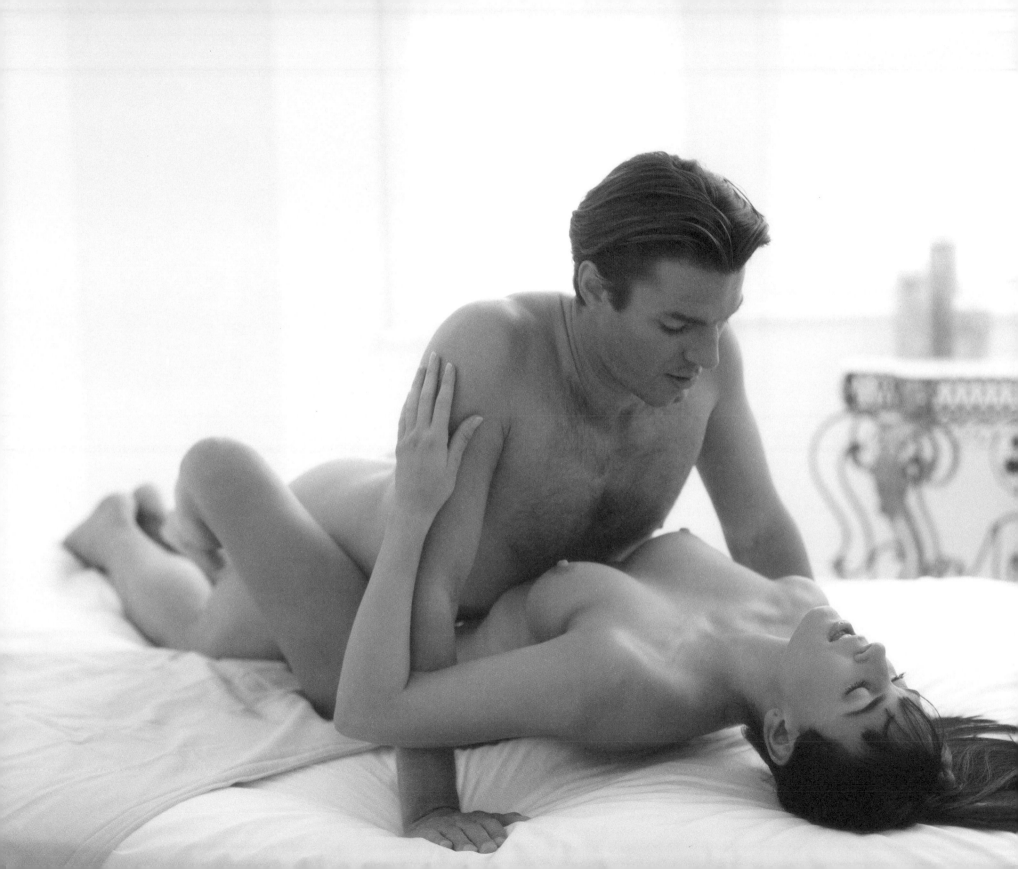

TANTRIC BREATH

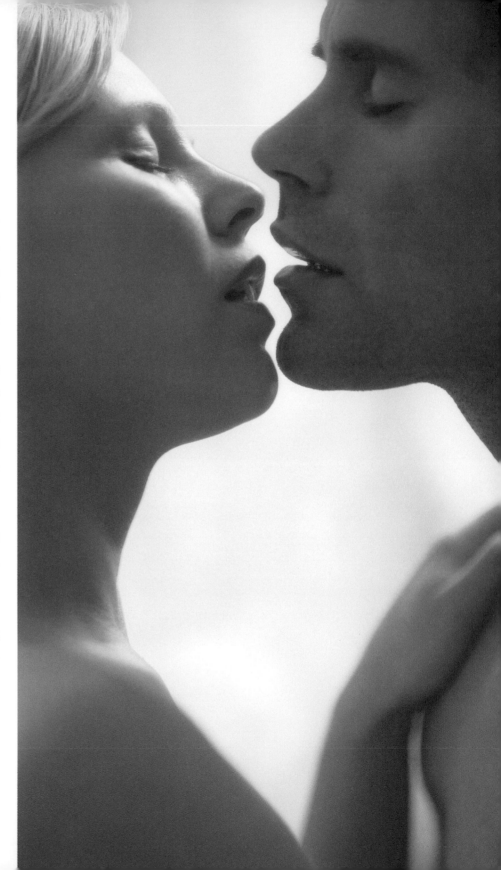

These Tantric breathing exercises deeply connect you to your partner. As you breathe with each other, you gradually get into an intoxicating rhythm that allows you to feel as though you are expanding beyond the physical limits of your bodies. These exercises are good preparation for the more advanced Tantric technique of Riding the Tiger (see pages 130–31).

Before attempting the breathing techniques, spend some time with your partner creating a sacred space (see pages 124–5) in which to practise. This helps you to feel as though you are about to do something special together. If you are feeling tense and want to unwind, do the yoga postures on pages 26–7.

BREATHING INTO THE HEART

Sit or kneel opposite your partner in your sacred space and look into each other's eyes. Now bring your attention to your breath and close your eyes. Imagine that you are breathing in through your genitals and drawing the breath all the way up to the level of your heart. As you exhale imagine the breath travelling back down your body and flowing out through your genitals. Don't try to do this in time with your partner yet, just concentrate on imagining your breath flowing from your genitals to your heart and back again – this alone takes practice.

Once you both feel confident, open your eyes, look at your partner and synchronize your breathing. Aim to match the pace and rhythm of each other's breath. Imagine that you are melting into one another.

ALTERNATE BREATHING

Sit or kneel opposite your partner in your sacred space and look into each other's eyes. Breathe deeply to start with (don't try to synchronize your breathing) and, when you feel ready, start to breathe alternately. She blows her breathe out in the direction of his lips and he inhales it. As she does this she imagines blowing love and energy into his body and he imagines drinking it in and letting it fill him with erotic feelings. Now as he breathes out, she drinks his breath into her body and feels permeated by loving energy. Think of the exercise as a way of making love to each other with your breath.

Once you can do this easily, imagine that as you inhale your partner's breath, you are pulling it all the way down through the centre of your body to your genitals. As you exhale, imagine the breath travelling all the way back up from your genitals and into your partner's mouth. Do this for around 5 minutes. You can enhance the feeling of connectedness by pressing your lips together and breathing directly into each other's mouths – if you do this you'll need to let in some fresh air from time to time.

As you breathe in and out of each other, cherish the experience of getting lost in the gentle rhythm of your breath.

FINISHING THE EXERCISES

When you finish any Tantric exercise it's important to allow yourself time to return to an ordinary state of being, especially if you encountered a state of expanded consciousness. Embrace or lie with your partner for as long as you want to. Then take some time to talk about your respective experiences – did you experience anything special? Did you find the techniques difficult? Did you feel self-conscious or were you able to let go?

THE *CHAKRAS*

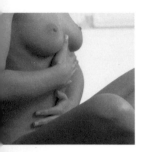

Anyone embarking on a Tantric path needs to have an awareness of the *chakras*: the seven wheels of energy that run along the central line of the body, from the base of the spine to the crown of the head. The *chakras* are part of our subtle anatomy; they can't usually be seen but, with practice, it's possible to become aware of the bodily sensations associated with each one.

THE SEVEN *CHAKRAS*

The first *chakra* is the base *chakra*. It lies on the perineum (between the anus and genitals) and is associated with the colour red, and basic physical survival. The second *chakra*, the belly *chakra*, lies over the spleen and is linked with the colour orange, and sexual energy and emotions. Next is the solar plexus *chakra* which lies over the navel – it is associated with the colour yellow, and issues of personal power.

The fourth *chakra* is the heart *chakra* in the centre of the chest. It is linked with the colour green, and love, care, compassion and devotion. The next two *chakras* are located at the throat and the brow (between the eyes). The throat *chakra* is connected with the colour blue; and with intuition, and the brow *chakra* with violet, and with the mind and psyche.

The seventh *chakra* is the crown *chakra* at the top of the head. This *chakra* is represented by white and is associated with spiritual enlightenment and connection to the divine.

THE AIM OF TANTRIC SEX

Through mindfulness (see pages 134–5) and specific practices (see pages 126–31) the Tantric student gradually learns how to harness sexual energy. As energy moves upward through each of the seven *chakras*, you attain a progressively higher level of consciousness. Ultimately, when energy reaches the crown *chakra*, you experience a blissful state of complete oneness and unity not only with your partner but with the entire universe.

Tantric practices are not a fast-track route to sexual connection and ecstasy with a lover. It takes time to become aware of the subtle body. An intellectual understanding of the subtle anatomy and the *chakra* system is no substitute for feeling the ecstatic sensations of energy rising and expanding inside you.

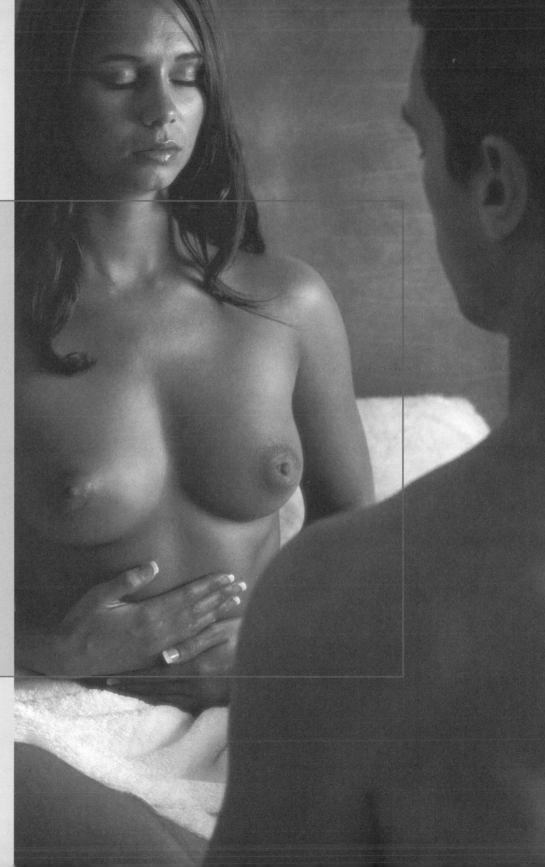

SENSUAL *CHAKRA* MEDITATION

Sit facing your partner in a comfortable position and synchronize your breathing. As you inhale deeply, imagine drawing up
red energy into your base *chakra* (see box, page 141). Let this
energy nurture your physical well-being.

The next time you breathe in, visualize the energy turning orange and flooding into your belly *chakra*. Concentrate on
feelings of eroticism. Breathe in again and let the energy turn
yellow and move up to your solar plexus *chakra* – explore any
powerful emotions you're holding onto, such as jealousy or
anger. Inhale and allow the energy to become green and ascend
to your heart centre. Focus on feelings of love for your partner.

Inhale and draw blue energy up to your throat *chakra* –
imagine this strengthening your intuition. As the energy turns
violet and moves up to your brow *chakra*, focus on your sense
of self. Finally, imagine white light moving to your crown *chakra*
and connecting you to everyone and everything around you.
Enjoy this sensation before allowing the white light to move
down through each of the *chakra*s, cleansing each one in turn.

RIDING THE TIGER

Riding the Tiger is a fairly advanced Tantric sex exercise that involves drawing energy up through your *chakras* one at a time as you make love. Before you try this, practise the *chakra* meditation on page 129 and the breathing exercises on pages 126–7.

STAGE ONE

Take turns to give each other an erotic massage (try the *lingam* and *yoni* massages on pages 18–21). When you both feel aroused and ready for penetration, he can sit in a Crossed-legged Position (see page 90) on the floor and she can sit on top of him and gently guide his penis into her vagina.

Now you need to synchronize your breathing and carefully balance your levels of arousal. You must remain sufficiently aroused for the penis to stay in the vagina but not so aroused that you ejaculate or have an orgasm. The aim of this exercise is to feel just close enough to orgasm so that you are able to direct sexual energy upward through your body instead of dissipating it outward. This takes practice to achieve so don't be disappointed if you feel you don't master the technique quickly.

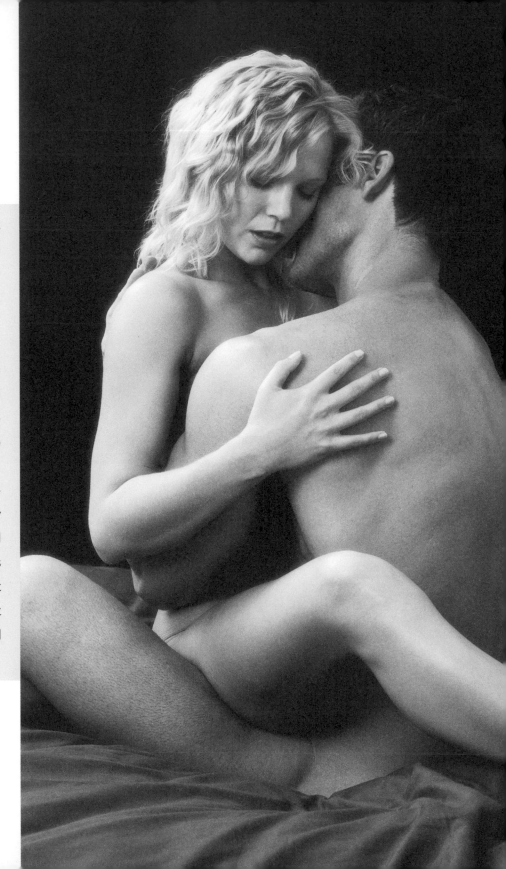

To maintain a balance of arousal, keep your movements small and subtle, and avoid thrusting. Squeeze your love muscles and rock your pelvis backward and forward. If this isn't arousing enough, go back to erotic massage until you feel ready for penetration again. If it's too stimulating, make smaller movements and focus on breathing together. Gaze into each other's eyes.

It is quite a leap to change the focus of lovemaking from big movements that lead to orgasm to small movements that keep you at the edge of orgasm. If you find stage one difficult, just stop here and discuss the sensations you each experienced.

STAGE TWO

Once you are on a plateau of arousal – near orgasm but not quite at the point of tipping over the edge into orgasm – work on building a rhythm together. As you inhale contract your love muscles, and as you exhale release the muscles (see pages 22–3). Practise this until you both achieve a natural rhythm.

Now as you inhale and contract your love muscles, imagine that you are drawing sexual energy (both your own and your partner's) up into your base *chakra* (see page 128). Hold your breath, then exhale and release your love muscles. Imagine the energy descending and leaving through your genitals. Do this several times and then try to draw the energy up to the belly and then the solar plexus *chakra*s. Visualize the energy as a warm, nourishing light. Imagine your partner's energy merging with yours. Immerse yourself in feelings rather than thoughts. Can you feel warm vibrations or a tingling spreading through your pelvis?

If you find it difficult to keep up the rhythm of breathing and muscle contraction while also visualizing the *chakra*s, take a break. You can return to the exercise on another occasion. When you feel comfortable with stage two, move on to stage three.

STAGE THREE

Keep practising the same rhythm, but try to draw energy up to the heart, throat, brow and crown *chakra*s. On each exhalation let the energy travel back down through the *chakra*s and out through your genitals. Finish this exercise with an embrace. When you feel ready, talk about the sensations you each experienced.

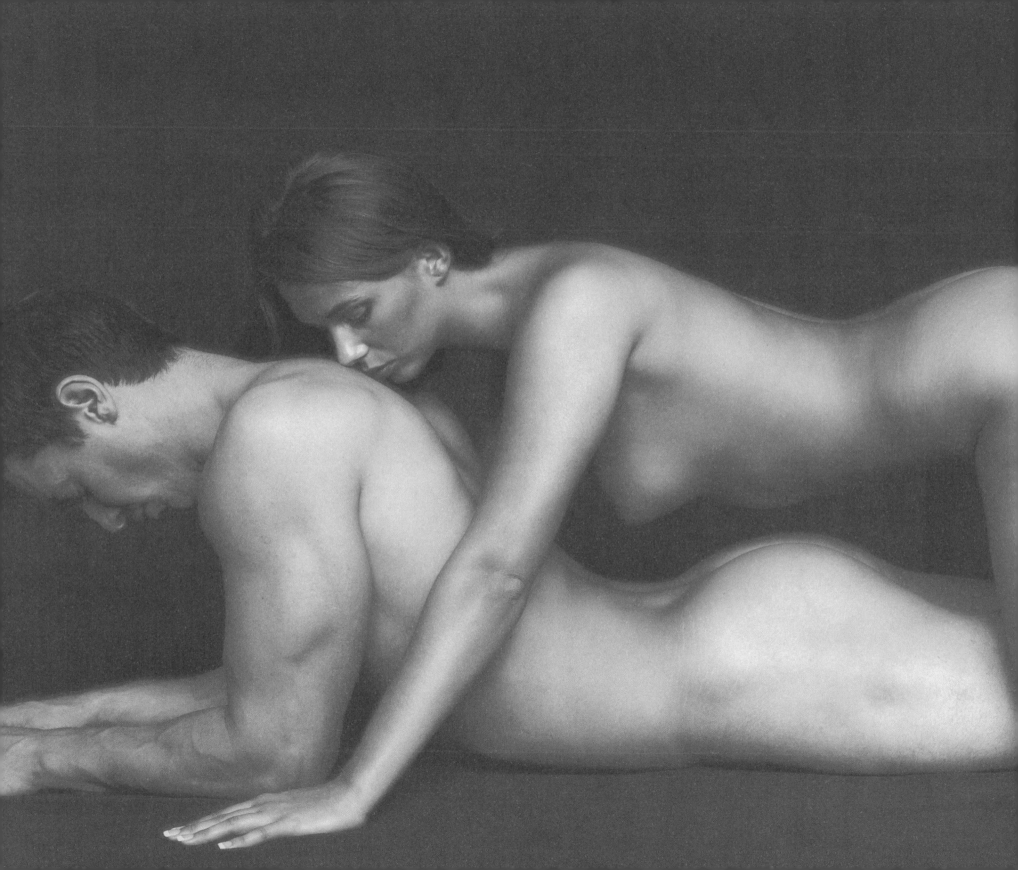

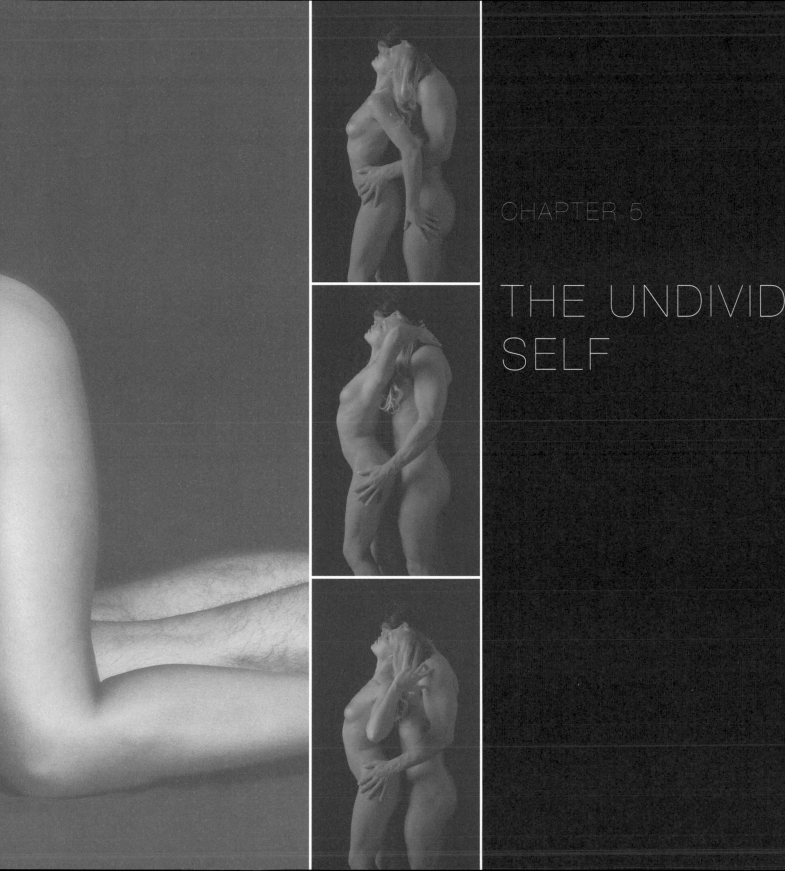

CHAPTER 5

THE UNDIVID
SELF

MINDFULNESS

Imagine how you feel at the absolute height of orgasm – for a brief moment you are completely immersed in blissful physical sensation, the world around you ceases to exist and you no longer know or care about time. Now imagine what it would be like if you could experience this sense of total absorption throughout sex – not just for the moment of climax but right from the first kiss to the post-sex cuddle.

VOICES IN YOUR HEAD

One of the problems many people experience during sex is a busy mind. Your body could be receiving the most expert stimulation imaginable, but if you're not mentally present, you won't experience the full joy of this. It's possible to be so accustomed to having a busy mind that you're not even aware of it. These are just some of the things it's common to think about during sex:

• Self-critical thoughts about your body. For example: "I look too fat when I take my clothes off."

• Critical thoughts about your or your partner's sexual performance. For example: "She doesn't seem to be enjoying this; what am I doing wrong?"

• Concern that you haven't got enough time for sex. For example: "I've got more important things I should be doing right now."

• Concern that you'll be interrupted. For example: "How long before the children come back?"

• Anxieties about making too much noise. For example: "I mustn't embarrass myself by moaning too loudly."

• Preoccupation with pressing issues at home or work. For example: "I can't relax until I've met that deadline."

• Anxieties about your emotional relationship with your partner. For example: "Have we got over that argument or is he still angry with me?"

The thoughts that cross your mind during sex don't even have to be negative – perhaps you spend time daydreaming. As one woman writes on the Internet: "Without any warning or logical connection to anything, my mind would take me to a square in Florence, a house in Greece, an outdoor hot-tub in Arizona, or a cliff overlooking the Pacific Ocean in California."

It doesn't matter what your mind is busy with; the fact is that you are thinking rather than feeling and this can take you away from the fullest possible experience of sex and intimacy. The first step is to recognize that you have a busy mind, identify what your thoughts are and then work toward mindfulness.

BEING IN THE MOMENT

Being present; being in the "now"; ecstasy; expanded consciousness; and peak experience: these are all different ways of describing mindfulness. To become mindful means to ignore the thoughts that flow through your mind and concentrate instead on the experiences that happen to you moment by moment. If your attention wanders you can gently but firmly draw it back by looking deeply into your lover's eyes or concentrating on the taste, smell, sounds and feelings of sex. Breathing in synchrony with your lover can also help you to become mindful. Signs of mindfulness include a sense of time slowing down (or forgetting about time), concentrating in a detailed way on the sensations of sex and feeling a sense of oneness with your lover.

PELVIC CIRCLING

Stand facing your lover and put your arms around each other. Spend a few moments enjoying the sensation of being held. Press the whole front surface of your body against your lover. This feels best if you're both naked and can feel the warm tactility of skin on skin. Now press your pelvis into your lover's pelvis – keep your arms wrapped around each other's body. Slowly begin to trace large circles with your joined pelvises. Breathe in slowly so that you complete your inhalation at the same time as you complete a full circle. Breathe out as you do the next circle, breathe in on the circle after that, and so on.

As well as synchronizing your inhalations and exhalations with the circular movements of your pelvises, you should also synchronize your breathing with each other. It may take a few rounds of circling to achieve this, but it will soon feel effortless and natural (see page 138). Try to relax into combined sensations of breathing and movement and allow yourself to get lost in them. See if you can experience a moment of peak connection with your lover.

LOVING KINDNESS

Have you ever felt that sex isn't what it used to be? If your sex life is flagging, it's worth looking at what's going on in your relationship. One of the main problems that can affect couples' sex lives is a slow but insidious build-up of resentment. Are you hanging on to negative feelings about each other? Do you have issues and arguments that have a long history and remain unresolved? Do you feel that your partner is able to listen to and understand you? An accumulation of negativity can gradually erode the strong sexual connection between lovers so that you have sex less often than you used to, or sex no longer feels as special or as satisfying.

DAY ZERO

One way of reconnecting is to dedicate a whole day to each other – think of it as "day zero". From day zero you will both pledge to relate to each other in a more open-hearted, generous and uncritical way. Make an effort to let go of lingering resentments and make a commitment to focus on the positive feelings that you have for each other rather than the negative

ones. Of course, this is easier said than done – couples with intractable problems may benefit from relationship counselling or sex therapy – but these techniques are a good way to start reawakening loving feelings.

Spend day zero doing things with and for each other. Give each other a massage (try the *yoni* and *lingam* massages on pages 18–21); prepare a delicious meal, go for a walk in a special or beautiful place; try the Tantric rituals on pages 120–27 or the Sensual Tour on pages 14–15; or play sex games and share your sexual fantasies (see pages 32–7).

If life with your partner has been difficult recently, reminisce about happier times. Talk about what you find attractive and sexy in each other. Be generous with your compliments – give them unconditionally without demanding that they be repaid. But, at the same time, mean what you say. Look into your partner's eyes as you speak. Resist the temptation to bring up old grievances and arguments – instead devote all of your mental energy to thinking of ways of making your partner feel fantastic. You will be the first to reap the rewards!

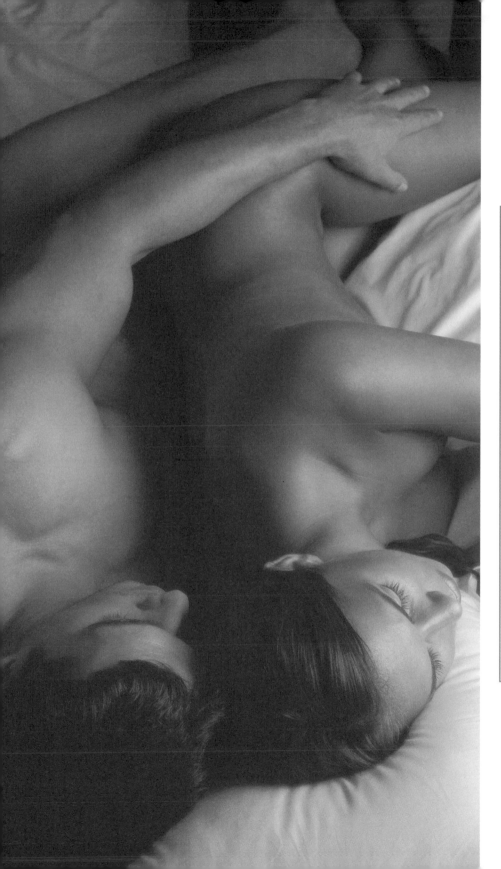

METTA BHAVANA

In Buddhism there is a meditation technique known as *metta bhavana*; *metta* means "love" and *bhavana* means "development". Here's an adapted version of the technique, which you can practise with your lover.

Sit on the floor opposite your lover in a crossed-legged position and concentrate on clearing your mind of negative energy. When you are feeling calm and centred, try to connect with the feelings of love and kindness that lie within you. To do this think of a time when you felt a powerful sense of love for either the person in front of you or someone else in your life. Relive the feelings that this love created and allow yourself to be filled by them. If this is difficult try this visualization: imagine your loving kindness as a jewel inside your body that is getting bigger and bigger and radiating warmth and light as it does so.

Now direct all your feelings of loving kindness toward your partner. Imagine that you are shining a light upon them. Look deeply into their eyes, cup their face in your hands and say "I love you".

BREATHE TOGETHER

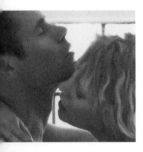

This technique for getting close to your lover is so obvious and simple that many couples overlook it. You don't need any tools or props. You don't need special lessons. You don't need to dress up or take roles. All you need is the power of your breath. The simple act of breathing in synchrony with your lover can take you to a timeless space where you both feel deeply connected.

SYNCHRONIZED BREATH

Sit or lie down together in a comfortable position. It can feel very intimate to lie with your faces touching or close (you can gaze into each other's eyes if you want to), but if you want to sit back-to-back or lie in the spoons position or another favourite position, that's fine too. Start by breathing normally and then after a couple of minutes begin to synchronize your breathing so that the length and texture of your inhalations and exhalations exactly match those of your partner. At first you may need to concentrate on making this happen, but after a few minutes it will start to come naturally. And you'll find that if your lover's breathing speeds up or slows down, yours will too.

Bring your entire awareness to the sound and sensation of the breath entering and leaving your and your partner's body. Let the everyday world drift away so that you can become fully absorbed in synchronous breathing. Make your breath as deep and smooth as you can – take the air deep into your belly. Feel all the boundaries between you and your partner melt away until the point where you have a sense of merging or "oneness". Some people find this exercise a joyous experience in which they imagine that they and their partner become a single breathing entity – the whole of their consciousness becomes tuned in to the simple ebb and flow of the breath.

SEXUAL TENSION

If you start to feel sexual tension mounting, let it gather momentum without acting upon it – keep the focus on your breathing. When you and your lover are very aroused and you both feel ready, slowly start to make love. Connecting in this way before sex will create a deep sense of trust and unity that ripples throughout your whole sexual encounter.

CONSCIOUS KISSING

Try this exercise in which you both promise to do nothing but kiss each other – for as long as possible. Stand close to your lover with your eyes closed and your lips almost touching. Breathe softly in and out so that your breath brushes each other's lips. Now gently graze the surface of his or her lips with yours before drawing your lover's lower lip into your mouth and caressing it with your lips and tongue (try experimenting with your teeth too). Explore the inside of your lover's mouth – as your kisses become more intimate, allow yourself to get carried away by them.

Don't think about what you're going to do next or whether or not kissing will lead to sex – just kiss for the sake of kissing. If your mind wanders, bring your attention back to the sensations in your body. Allow your senses to open up so that you really begin to relish the taste, smell and feel of your lover's lips and tongue against yours. Lose yourself in the act of kissing – the more absorbed you become in the experience, the more deeply connected you will become to your lover.

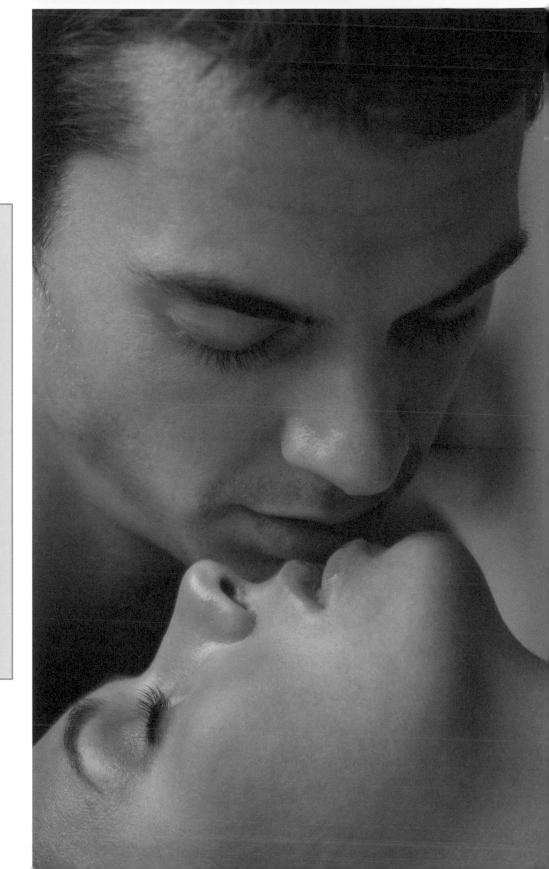

CREATIVE VISUALIZATION

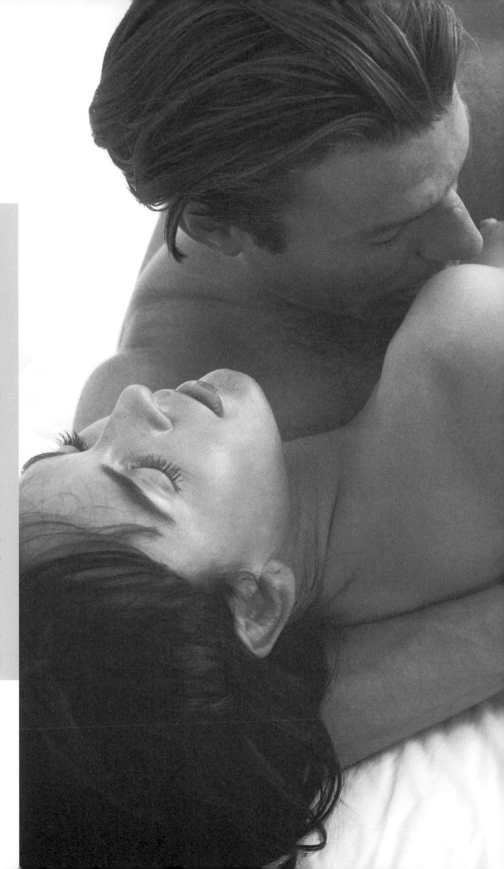

Creating strong sexual images in your mind can boost your arousal, your sexual confidence, the pleasure you experience during sex and even the intensity of your orgasms. For some people visualization comes very naturally, for others it is elusive – but most of us can develop our visual imagination with practice.

MIND MOVIES

The Tantric sex writer Margot Anand recommends the following technique for visualization. Lie down and breathe deeply. As you begin to relax, imagine that behind your eyelids is a blank screen onto which you can project any image you like – even a movie. Allow sexual images to come to the forefront of your mind and project them onto your screen. Embellish the images with as much detail as you can. For example, if you are fantasizing about two strangers making love, imagine the room they are in, the way the light falls on their bodies, their facial expressions and so on. Be really specific about what you "see" – even down to the beads of sweat on the small of his back or the way she moves her hips. Bring your visualization alive by imagining sounds and smells as well as sights. These visualizations can be the product of your own invention or they can be memories of previous sexual experiences, or erotic scenes from movies.

PRACTISING VISUALIZATION

Men are particularly responsive to visual cues during sex. He can enhance his arousal by visualizing images that he finds titillating – his lover undressing, lying naked in bed or caressing herself. If he finds himself becoming distracted during sex or worrying about his performance, he can choose a powerful image – a close-up of his penis moving in and out of her vagina or her lips and tongue caressing his penis – to project onto his mental movie screen.

Some women find it difficult to become aroused or to reach orgasm, but a really hot mental image can tip her over the edge. She can build up an image bank of mental pictures that have the power to turn her on. She can try imagining what his fingers or tongue look like as they caress her clitoris, or his erect penis as he ejaculates. If genitally-focused images don't work for her, she can replay the events of a favourite fantasy in her mind.

BOOSTING AROUSAL

Before you have sex, try this visualization to send your arousal levels sky high. Take off your clothes, close your eyes and ask your lover to read the following instructions to you.

Sit down in a crossed-legged position or sit with one of your heels pressed against your genitals. Concentrate on the gentle pressure produced by the floor or your heel. Alternatively, you can press the palm of your hand lightly against your genitals. Breathe slowly and let your body relax.

As you inhale imagine that you are drawing up sexual energy through your genitals (in the same way that the roots of a plant draw up water). This energy feels hot and tingling. Imagine that it is a deep, rich red colour. Each time you inhale, imagine that you are drawing up more of this red sexual energy. Visualize it spreading and blossoming throughout your genitals and pelvis – this whole area is becoming increasingly hot and sensitive. If this feels good let your entire body fill up with sexual energy until your whole interior feels as though it is tingling and vibrating with pleasure.

THE RHYTHM OF SEX

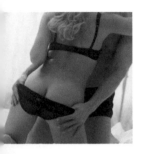

Have you ever noticed how you can have really hot sex one night and yet just a couple of days later, sex isn't even lukewarm? All of us have sexual "hot times" that depend upon a complex interaction of factors: hormone levels, biorhythms, fatigue, stress and how connected you feel to one another. Here's how to spot the hot times so that you can exploit them to the max.

THE POWER OF HORMONES

Libido is driven by the male hormone testosterone. In women testosterone is produced by the ovaries and the adrenal glands, and levels peak around the time of ovulation. Some women also feel the libido-boosting effects of testosterone most strongly just before or during menstruation. In men testosterone levels peak first thing in the morning — so if you and your lover are both morning people, this is a great time to make love. However, male testosterone levels may also fluctuate in cycles.

You and your partner can try keeping a "sex diary". Note the times at which you feel most sexy (record any increases in masturbation and intercourse and also sexual dreams, thoughts and fantasies). If your hot times occur in unison, make a note of this and clear your schedule for sex!

DAILY HIGHS AND LOWS

All of us experience peaks and troughs in our levels of emotional, intellectual and physical well-being and these are the result of biorhythms. The most well-researched type of biorhythm is the circadian rhythm — a 24-hour biological cycle during which energy levels go up and down. Most of us either feel more awake and energized in the morning or in the evening. If you are a morning person and you habitually have sex last thing at night, you can breathe new life into sex simply by making love at a different time of day. Alternatively, if you do have sex in the evening, wake yourself up beforehand by going for a brisk walk.

Relationships also go through highs and lows. If you're experiencing a low, your sex life may suffer. If there's discord in your relationship, try doing the loving-kindness exercises on pages 136–7 or Tantric rituals on pages 120–27. The closer you feel to your lover the hotter the sex!

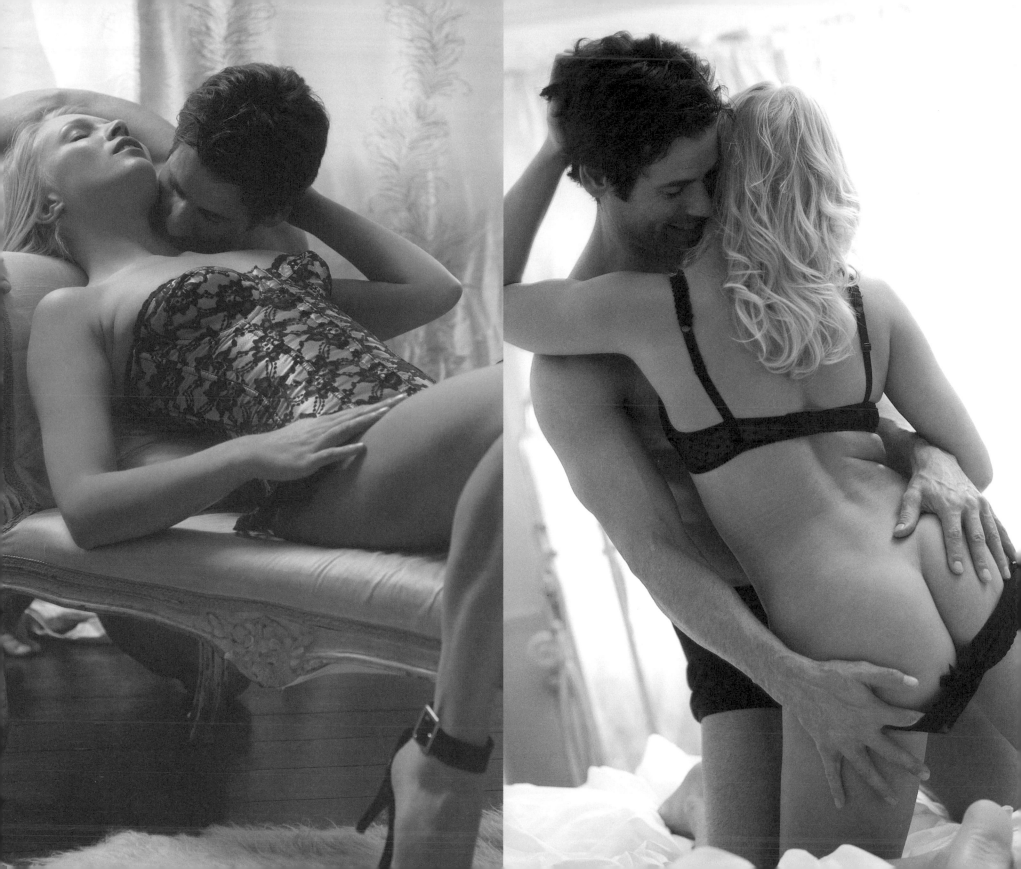

SEX WITHOUT GOALS

If you're bored with old sexual habits and you want to learn new ways to please your lover, then this sex therapy program is a great way to learn how to stimulate each other. The program lasts 12 days (these can be spread over two, three or more weeks rather than being consecutive days). Although it may seem counterintuitive, the program demands that you abstain from sexual intercourse until the very end. The point of this is not to make you feel sex-starved, but to force your attention away from the "goals" of penetration and orgasm and toward the delights of sensual and playful touch.

DAYS 1–3

Spend around 15 to 30 minutes a day touching and stroking your partner's naked body. For ideas about new ways of touching, read the Sensual Tour on pages 14–15. Try to make your touches sensual rather than directly sexual – avoid erogenous areas such as the genitals and nipples. Aim to make your partner's hair stand on end with pleasure. Now swap and let your partner touch and stroke your naked body. The aim is to explore and experiment with subtle forms of touch, rather than to turn each other on. If you do get aroused, that's OK, but you should avoid having intercourse.

DAYS 4–6

Spend 15 to 30 minutes a day touching and stroking your partner's naked body, but this time you're going to include their genitals and nipples. To prevent you touching your lover in familiar places and habitual ways, pretend that you've never touched your lover before and that you must learn to stimulate them for the first time (some people find this easier if they wear a blindfold). Use your lips, tongue, fingers, hair or feet as massage tools – there are no rules about what you can and can't do. Now swap with your partner. Give each other plenty of feedback – if you like you can use a rating system. Award a "5" for something that feels wonderful and a lower score for something that feels less good. It's also fine to give your partner instructions such as "harder", "softer", "slower" or "faster". Don't aim to give each other an orgasm; as before, avoid intercourse.

DAYS 7–8

Repeat the previous stage of the program, but this time try using massage oils and genital lubricants. Apply some warm oil to your partner's skin so that your hands glide smoothly against their body. And use slow sensual strokes to apply oil or lubricant to your partner's genitals – after at least a week of abstaining from sex, this can be instantaneously erotic! But remember to keep exploring the whole of each other's body – it's very easy to just focus on each other's genitals, because these are the hot spots of sensation. Continue to avoid using habitual techniques that you've used in the past (even if they bring results). Your aim is to learn new ways of touching.

DAYS 9–11

At this point of the program you can stop taking turns with your partner and start touching each other at the same time. Spend 15 to 30 minutes a day touching and stroking each other's naked body. Use oils if this feels good. Tell each other if you really enjoy something. Just one more day until you can have sex!

DAY 12

This is the final day of the program and your aim is to integrate all the new techniques you've learned to give each other an orgasm and to have intercourse. Keep sex slow and sensual and make it a whole-body experience that incorporates all of your lover's erogenous zones from the crown of their head to the soles of their feet. Orgasm can happen during intercourse or independently of it – be creative.

DEBRIEFING

After you and you partner have completed the sex program, talk to each other in detail about your experiences. Was it hard not having sex until the 12th day? Do you feel that slowing down your approach to sex was useful? Did you discover erogenous zones that you didn't know you had? Do you feel that sex can now be more exciting and less predictable than it used to be? Have you made any surprising discoveries about each other? Discuss the possibility of repeating the program at regular intervals (perhaps twice a year) to reinvigorate your sex life.

POST-COITAL CONNECTION

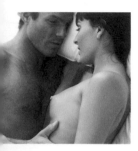

Good sex is an exhilarating experience that you both need time to "come down" from. This means lying together and soaking up the experience that you've just shared. Now is not the time for sexual postmortems or dissecting what went right or wrong.

According to *The Perfumed Garden*, post-coital behaviour may even influence conception: if the man gently withdraws from the woman as she lies on her right side, then the chances of conceiving a son are increased. *The Perfumed Garden* also advises couples to rest, refrain from rigorous exercise and avoid drinking rain water (which is said to weaken the loins) after sex!

ENJOY THE SEX HIGH

People think of orgasm as the high point of sex, but the aftermath can be just as good in a more diffused and sensual kind of way. Enjoy basking in the post-sex cocktail of feel-good chemicals known as endorphins and oxytocin. Endorphins are released during sex, exercise and labour – they are the body's natural painkillers and they induce drug-like feelings of bliss. Oxytocin is released during sex and after childbirth and is known as the "cuddle chemical" because it gives you that warm glow that comes from feeling intimate and bonded with another person.

THE WIND-DOWN PHASE

If you have to get up to continue with your day after sex, allow yourself at least 10 to 15 minutes so that your body can slowly return to its pre-aroused state. Sexologists Masters and Johnson call this stage of sex the "resolution phase". In it your heartbeat, breathing rate and blood pressure return to normal and the blood flows away from the genitals. While these changes take place, you can enter a relaxed state by lying close together and breathing in synchrony. As long as your lover doesn't feel left behind, let yourself float off into a delicious and dreamy sleep.

Sexual pleasure doesn't have to end when intercourse does. The post-coital period is a great time for a woman who hasn't come during intercourse – her lover can give undivided attention to her clitoris and vagina. Depending on a man's refractory period (the length of time it takes for him to regain his erection), you can also make love several times in a row.

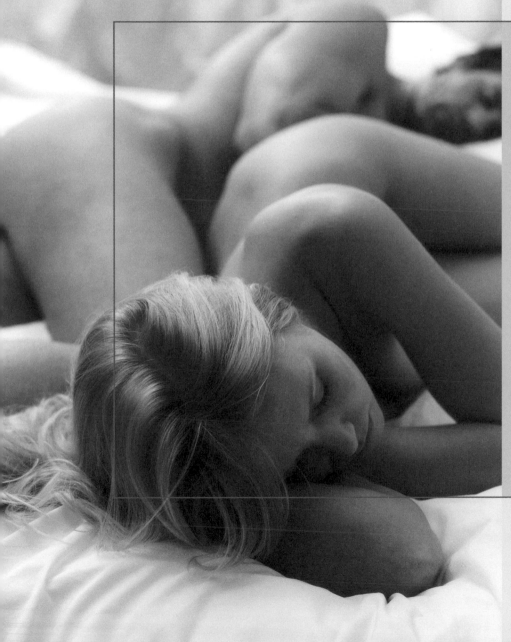

POST-SEX POSITIONS

There's a unique specialness about the moments after sex, and nurturing them is a great way to feel really close to one another. Kiss each other gently, be reverent, whisper how much you love your partner and stroke each other's face or body. Here are four intimate positions in which to enjoy the post-sex come-down.

The Spoons Position: you both lie on your sides, his back to her belly (or vice versa), nestled into one another like two spoons.

Contrary Position (see page 85): she lies on top of his body with his penis still inside her vagina (but don't do this if he is wearing a condom; as the penis becomes soft the condom will be more likely to slip off).

Side-by-side Clasping Position (see page 57): you and your lover lie on your sides facing each other and looking deeply into each other's eyes.

Thigh Clasp (see page 80): you lie on your sides facing one another with her thighs wrapped around his body (if he's heavy, she can just wrap her upper thigh around him).

SEXUAL INSPIRATION

Keeping the sexual spark alive in a relationship takes work. Whether you're into Tantric sex, bondage or gentle massage, sex needs to be nurtured. If you feel that your relationship needs an injection of passion, rise to the challenge – make the search for sexual inspiration into your most pressing project.

DO IT DIFFERENTLY

If you're bored with making love in the same old way, do the opposite. If you have sex with the lights on, turn them off. If you make love in the bedroom, do it in the dining room. If you go to bed naked, start wearing erotic lingerie. If you have a set sequence of moves, change it. If you habitually close your eyes, open them and gaze at each other. If you both come quickly, try the peaking technique in which you repeatedly bring each other to the edge of orgasm and then withdraw stimulation. Only allow your lover to climax when they can't take being teased for a second longer. Don't forget to seduce you partner: write them sexy or provocative notes or text messages, flirt with them – make them feel like the sexiest person alive.

SEX HOMEWORK

Make a list of all the things you'd like to try with your lover and playfully present this list to them as "sex homework". Here are some suggestions.

- Throw a surprise party – just the two of you, a bed and a bottle of champagne on ice.
- Turn out the lights and explore each other's body by candlelight.
- Spend an entire day together naked.
- Paint each other with body paint.
- Role-play at being a sexual servant for the evening.
- Strip to music.
- Buy a sex toy that you've never used before.
- Read each other erotic bedtime stories.
- Play naked hide-and-seek.
- Make a sexual toy box.
- Take sexy pictures of each other using an instant camera.
- Play some sensual music and seduce each other by dancing erotically together.

BECOME A SEXPERT

Don't believe that you know everything about sex or even everything sexual about your lover. Treat sex as a voyage of discovery that you are making together. If you are interested in Tantric sex, go on a course. Read books about sex and about other peoples' experience of sex. Men can find out about women's sexuality by reading books such as *The Hite Report* by Shere Hite and women can find out about men's sexuality by reading books such as *Men in Love* by Nancy Friday. (Details for both these books can be found on page 150.)

If there's an aspect of sex that arouses your curiosity, such as fetishism, explore it. Dress up, take on roles, watch erotic movies with your partner – or make your own. Throw a sex-themed party in which guests have to dress up as their favourite sexual fantasy. Above all, talk about your experiences and fantasies so that you really know what makes each other tick sexually. Talking about sex is often a prelude to having sex.

The Internet has transformed the way we access information about sex; new ideas to try out in bed are now just a click away. Surf the Internet with your lover talking about the things that turn you on – and the things that don't. Many couples find this experience both liberating and inspiring. Not all sex sites are hard-core, many are erotic rather than pornographic, and plenty are designed to educate and inform.

MAKE YOUR RELATIONSHIP WORK

Strong, healthy relationships form the basis for good sex, so dedicate time to making sure that you and your partner feel good together. If you feel your relationship is struggling, make it a priority to resolve problems now, either through talking to each other or seeking professional help from a therapist. Cultivating intimacy means spending uninterrupted time alone together, talking about the things you feel are important, and listening generously and impartially when it's your partner's turn to talk. Keep romance alive in your relationship by remembering what first attracted you to one another and what you love and value in each other now. And remember that sex is one of the best celebrations of love there is.

FURTHER READING

Amoda, Jivan *Moving into Ecstasy* (HarperCollins, London and Thorsons, New York, 2001)

Anand, Margot *The New Art of Sexual Ecstasy* (HarperCollins, London and Thorsons, New York, 2003)

Burton, Sir Richard F. and Arbuthnot, Forster F. (translators) *The Illustrated Kama Sutra, Ananga Ranga, Perfumed Garden* (Hamlyn, London, 1987 and Park Street Press, Vermont, USA, 1991)

Comfort, Alex *The Joy of Sex/ The Joy of Sex: Fully Revised and Completely Updated for the 21st Century* (Mitchell Beazley, London, 1996 and Crown, New York, 2002)

Doniger, Wendy and Kakar, Sudhir (translators) *Kamasutra* (Oxford University Press, Oxford, 2002 and USA, 2003)

Fraser, Tara *Yoga for You* (UK)/*Total Yoga* (US) (Duncan Baird Publishers, London and Thorsons, New York, 2001)

Friday, Nancy *Forbidden Flowers: More Women's Sexual Fantasies* (Arrow, London, 1994 and Pocket Books, New York, 1993)

Friday, Nancy *Men in Love* (Arrow, London, 1980 and Delta, New York, 1998)

Friday, Nancy *My Secret Garden* (Quartet Books, London, 1979 and Pocket Books, New York, 1998)

Friday, Nancy *Women on Top* (Arrow, London and Pocket Books, New York, 1993)

Hite, Shere *The New Hite Report* (Hamlyn, London, 2000 and Seven Stories Press, New York, 2003)

Hooper, Anne *Pure Sex* (Duncan Baird Publishers, London and Thorsons, New York, 2003)

Hooper, Anne *The Body Electric* (HarperCollins, London, 1984)

Lorius, Cassandra *101 Nights of Tantric Sex* (Thorsons, London, 2002 and New York, 2003)

Love, Patricia and Robinson, Jo *Hot Monogamy* (Piatkus, London, 1998 and Plume, New York, 1999)

Masters, William H. et al *Human Sexuality* (Pearson, London, 1995 and Addison-Wesley, Boston, 1995)

Ray Stubbs, Kenneth *Kama Sutra of Sexual Positions, The Tantric Art of Love* (Rider, London and Penguin Putnam, New York, 2003)

Ray Stubbs, Kenneth et al *Tantric Massage: The Erotic Touch of Love* (UK)/ *Erotic Massage: The Tantric Touch of Love* (US) (Rider, London, 2004 and Penguin Putnum, New York, 1999)

Smith, Karen *Massage: The Power of Healing Touch* (Duncan Baird Publishers, London, 1998 and Thorsons, New York, 2003)

Winks, Cathy *The Good Vibrations Guide: The G-Spot* (Down There Press, San Francisco, 1999)

INDEX

ACKNOWLEDGMENTS
Author's acknowledgments
Thanks to Zoë, Jules and Manisha at Duncan Baird. Thanks also to Mark O'Connor.

Models for commissioned photography supplied by International Model Management (IMM), London

John Davis is represented by Gina Phillips